Published and forthcoming Oxford American Handbooks

Oxford American Handbook of Anesthesiology
Oxford American Handbook of Clinical Dentistry
Oxford American Handbook of Clinical Medicine
Oxford American Handbook of Surgery
Oxford American Handbook of Critical Care
Oxford American Handbook of Emergency Medicine
Oxford American Handbook of Otolaryngology
Oxford American Handbook of Nephrology and Hypertension
Oxford American Handbook of Obstetrics and Gynecology
Oxford American Handbook of Pediatrics
Oxford American Handbook of Psychiatry
Oxford American Handbook of Pulmonary Medicine

OXFORD MEDICAL PUBLICATIONS

Oxford American Handbook of
Otolaryngology

Oxford American Handbook of **Otolaryngology**

Andrew Blitzer, MD, DDS

Professor of Clinical Otolaryngology
College of Physicians and Surgeons of
Columbia University

Jerome S. Schwartz, MD

Voluntary Clinical Faculty
Georgetown University Hospital Center
Washington, DC
Clinical Otolaryngologist
Feldman ENT, P.C.

Phillip C. Song

Division of Laryngology
Massachusetts Eye and Ear Infirmary
Instructor in Otology and Laryngology
Harvard Medical School

Nwanmegha Young, MD

Assistant Professor of Surgery
Section of Otolaryngology
Yale School of Medicine

with

Rogan Corbridge

Nicholas Steventon

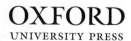

OXFORD
UNIVERSITY PRESS

OXFORD
UNIVERSITY PRESS

Oxford University Press, Inc., publishes works that further
Oxford University's objective of excellence
in research, scholarship, and education.

Oxford New York

Auckland Cape Town Dar es Salaam Hong Kong Karachi
Kuala Lumpur Madrid Melbourne Mexico City Nairobi
New Delhi Shanghai Taipei Toronto

With offices in

Argentina Austria Brazil Chile Czech Republic France Greece
Guatemala Hungary Italy Japan Poland Portugal Singapore
South Korea Switzerland Thailand Turkey Ukraine Vietnam

Copyright © 2008 by Oxford University Press, Inc.

Published by Oxford University Press, Inc.
198 Madison Avenue, New York, New York 10016

www.oup.com

Oxford is a registered trademark of Oxford University Press

Library of Congress Cataloging-in-Publication Data
Oxford American handbook of otolaryngology/Andrew Blitzer ... [et al.].
p. ; cm. — (Oxford American handbooks)
Based on: Oxford handbook of ENT and head and neck surgery/Rogan
Corbridge and Nicholas Steventon. 2006.
Includes bibliographical references and index.
ISBN 978-0-19-534337-3
1. Otolaryngology—Handbooks, manuals, etc.
2. Head—Surgery—Handbooks, manuals, etc. 3. Neck—Surgery—Handbooks,
manuals, etc. I. Blitzer, Andrew. II. Corbridge, Rogan J. Oxford
handbook of ENT and head and neck surgery. III. Title: Handbook of
otolaryngology. IV. Series.
[DNLM: 1. Otorhinolaryngologic Diseases—Handbooks.
2. Head—surgery—Handbooks. 3. Neck—surgery—Handbooks.
4. Otorhinolaryngologic Surgical Procedures—Handbooks. WV 39 O98 2008]
RF56.O94 2008
617.5'1—dc22   2007044670

9 8 7 6 5 4 3 2 1

Printed in China
on acid-free paper

Preface

This book is intended for the medical student, physician-in-training, or Otolaryngology resident, or as a quick reference for the practitioner of Otolaryngology. This volume is not meant to be encyclopedic, since the breadth of Otolaryngology knowledge is so large.

Instead, it is meant to be a pocket book that can be an easy reference for the student or practitioner. It covers common otolaryngologic disorders and is organized by anatomic site, disease entity, presentation, or procedure. Current references are included for further reading and more in-depth information. It is hoped that physicians and surgeons at all levels will find this book valuable.

The authors would like to thank Kevin Kochanski, William Lamsback, and Nancy Wolitzer, our developmental editors at Oxford University Press, for all of their assistance in organizing this volume, and David Cognetti and Berrylin Ferguson for their help in editing the manuscript. In addition, we are indebted to Myung Song of Woodstock, New York, for her medical illustrations in Chapter 16, on facial plastic surgery and reconstruction.

Contents

Detailed contents

Overview

Using this book

The purpose of this book is to provide concise, practical guidelines associated with treating disorders of the head and neck. We wish to provide a basic fund of knowledge of Otolaryngology, with particular emphasis on common ear, nose, and throat (ENT) problems. The breadth of Otolaryngology practice is so wide today that an attempt to be comprehensive would be impossible, and for the sake of brevity, many of the subtleties of clinical practice have been excluded here. As a reference book, the Oxford Handbook is well organized and designed to be slipped inside the pocket of a white coat for rapid consultation. It is suitable for the ward, rounds, and clinic. In addition, we have included reference lists at the end of each chapter that provide a more in-depth understanding of each disorder.

The book is organized as a primer to Otolaryngology. It begins with a description of the head and neck examination and history taking as related to disorders of the head and neck. Unique for this type of book is Chapter 3, "Common methods of presentation," which is a guide for dealing with patients as they present with symptoms in clinical practice. It also provides a convenient way of accessing the relevant chapter in the anatomical list. The bulk of the handbook is organized on the basis of anatomic sites. The last several chapters are very helpful for describing common surgical procedures used in Otolaryngology, ENT emergencies, and common eponyms used.

Otolaryngology as a subject and career

Otolaryngology is a fantastic specialty that is every bit as exciting in practice as it is in theory. It is difficult to conceive of any specialty that can provide such diversity in medical practice.

- ENT conditions make up 25%–50% of all general-practice consultations.
- ENT conditions affect people of all ages, from infants to the elderly.
- Outpatient work is about 50% of the workload. This gives a good balance between surgical and medical practice.
- The major broad divisions of Otolaryngology and head and neck surgery include otology and neurotology, rhinology, facial plastics and reconstructive surgery, head and neck cancer surgery, laryngology, allergy, and pediatric Otolaryngology.
- Surgical skills are broad, from microsurgery on the smallest bones in the body to major head and neck reconstructive surgery.
- Otolaryngology offers enormous research potential, including nasal polyps, congenital hearing loss, immunology, and genetics of cancer.
- Cutting-edge developments are occurring in Otolaryngology, such as cochlear implantation, auditory brainstem implantation, and laser surgery. There is a constant evolution of surgical techniques and devices.

Further sources of information

- American Academy of Otolaryngology and Head and Neck Surgery
  www.entnet.org
- American Academy of Facial Plastic and Reconstructive Surgery
  www.aafprs.org
- American Broncho-Esophagological Association
  www.abea.net
- American Society of Pediatric Otolaryngologists
  www.aspo.us
- American Laryngological Association
  www.alahns.org
- The Triological Society
  www.triological.org
- American Neurotology Society
  www.americanneurotologysociety.com
- American Academy of Otolaryngic Allergy
  www.aaoaf.org
- American Rhinologic Society
  www.american-rhinologic.org

Students and Otolaryngology

The subject of Otolaryngology can seem quite daunting to students. This vast subject occupies a small part of the medical curriculum, and in some instances has been dropped entirely from medical-school programs.

In strong contrast to the time given to the field in training, otolaryngological conditions make up between 25% and 50% of all general-practice consultations. As a student, it is important to have a firm idea of the important topics you want to cover in Otolaryngology. These will form your learning aims and objectives—see the next section (p. 5). There may be local variations.

Although you will find that Otolaryngology departments throughout the world are welcoming to students, do not abuse their hospitality by being late or discourteous. Professional conduct is important, whatever the specialty you are studying.

There are particularly sensitive areas within Otolaryngology practice that require special tact as a student. Two of these are head and neck cancer and hearing problems.

Head and neck cancer

These cancers form an important part of the Otolaryngology workload. You will need to be sensitive in dealing with these patients. They often have unique problems associated with their disease and treatment including the following:
- Poor communication
- Disfiguring surgery
- Depression
- Alcohol withdrawal

Hearing problems

The diagnosis of hearing loss in a child can be a devastating blow to parents. You will need to be sensitive to this. Another cause of great concern to parents is when a poorly performing child has a normal hearing test, as this may confirm the diagnosis of global developmental delay.

ENT learning aims and objectives for clinical medical students

Aims

- To acquire sufficient knowledge of ENT conditions to be able to recognize common problems and when and what to refer
- To understand that ENT conditions are extremely common and form a large part of the workload of a general practitioner
- To learn the skills required to examine patients with ENT diseases and to make a presumptive diagnosis
- To learn how to prioritize and manage different ENT conditions
- To become stimulated by and interested in the specialty of Otolaryngology

Objectives

- To learn the signs and symptoms of common ENT conditions
- To learn the techniques of ear, nasal, and neck examination
- To demonstrate an understanding of the basic anatomy and physiology of the ear and upper aerodigestive tract, and relate this knowledge to the signs and symptoms of ENT disease
- To understand the medical and surgical treatment of common ENT conditions
- To be familiar with the commonly used medications for treating ENT problems, and their side effects
- To understand the risks and complications of surgery
- To recognize the different ways in which head and neck malignancy can present, and to understand that early diagnosis of head and neck cancer leads to improved survival
- To learn the ways in which ENT-related communication difficulties can arise and be overcome
- To appreciate and be sensitive to the impact of ENT conditions on patients and their families

Student Otolaryngology curriculum

Practical skills

- Use of the otoscope to examine the external auditory meatus and tympanic membrane
- Basic examination of the nose
- Examination of the oral cavity and oropharynx
- Examination of the neck
- Management of a nosebleed
- Dealing with a tracheotomy

Ear

- Basic anatomy and physiology of the ear
- Presentation and management of common ear disease, e.g., otitis externa, otitis media, glue ear, chronic suppurative otitis media with or without cholesteatoma, vertigo, and facial palsy
- Examination of the ear, including that of the pinna and ear canal, and otoscopy
- Testing of hearing with tuning fork tests
- Advantages of the microscope and the fiberoptic otoscope
- Basic interpretation of audiometry, pure-tone audiograms, and tympanograms
- Principles of grommet insertion, mastoid surgery, and treatment of Menieres disease
- Identification of postoperative problems following ear surgery, i.e., sensorineural hearing loss, facial nerve palsy, and vestibular dysfunction
- Understanding the differential diagnosis of facial nerve palsy and its treatment

Nose

- Anatomy and physiology of the nose
- Symptoms and signs of common sinonasal disease, e.g., rhinitis, sinusitis, nasal polyps
- Examination of the nose, including assessment of the appearance, the septum, the turbinates, and the mucosa
- Endoscopic evaluation of the nose
- Management of a fractured nose and the timing of intervention
- Management of epistaxis, from minor nosebleeds to torrential hemorrhage
- Principles of common nasal operations, including septal surgery, functional endoscopic sinus surgery, and rhinoplasty

Head and neck—benign and malignant disease

- Basic anatomy and physiology of the oral cavity, salivary glands, pharynx, larynx, esophagus, and lymph node drainage
- Presentation of head and neck cancer
- Presentation and management of salivary gland disease
- Examination of the oral cavity, larynx, and pharynx, including use of the endoscope
- Examination of the neck with reference to the lymph nodes
- The role of fine needle aspiration cytology (FNAC)
- Principles and limitations of radiological investigation of the head and neck region
- Management of neck masses, in particular the malignant lymph node with an unknown primary
- Management of the airway in patients with a tracheotomy or end tracheostomy after laryngectomy
- A basic knowledge of the principles of operative surgery, in particular the principles of reconstructive surgery and the surgery for salivary gland disease, e.g., parotidectomy
- Postoperative management of a patient who has undergone major head and neck surgery
- The role of the multidisciplinary team in head and neck cancer and voice disorders

Supplementary knowledge

- The role of otoacoustic emissions and evoked auditory potentials in managing hearing loss
- Use of speech audiometry
- Surgery for otosclerosis
- Bone-anchored hearing aids for conductive hearing loss
- Cochlear implantation and reactions of the deaf community to this intervention
- Neuro-otology, in particular the presentation and management of acoustic neuromas
- Craniofacial surgery and the interplay between Otolaryngology, plastic surgery, and neurosurgery
- Management of cleft palate
- Advanced endoscopic sinus surgery for mangement of sinonasal malignancy, pituitary tumors, and skull base tumors
- Microlaryngeal surgery and surgical voice restoration
- Use of chemotherapy and radiotherapy in head and neck malignancy

Research

In conducting research, it is important to learn how to ask a question, establish a hypothesis and test it, and develop a database and conclusions based on statistically sound results. Aim to produce at least one publication every 6 months. Don't be distracted by trying to be involved in too many projects at once.

Work in a team if you can, as collaboration is a valuable component to your education. Don't take on too many projects in a team—each team member should take on one research project at a time. Ask senior colleagues about possible projects; affiliated university departments may be helpful in this regard. Involve a statistician before undertaking research, as this will often help turn an idea into a first-rate publication and avoid unnecessary work. Always check local ethics committee guidelines before you start.

Critical appraisal of the literature

Staying current and up to date in medical care requires the ability to critically appraise the literature and to understand the methodology required to produce clinically significant work. More clinical decisions are being evaluated by outcomes and tested by clinical trials. Evidence-based medicine (EBM) is based on the application of results of prospective, controlled studies. It is important to understand the level of evidence supported by our clinical decisions. Studies should be judged on both internal validity (is the methodology used by the researchers valid?) and external validity (does the study answer the question that you are asking?).

Questions to ask when assessing the strength of a clinical study:

1. How were the patients recruited, and what is the setting in which the study took place?
2. Are the inclusion criteria appropriate and free of bias?
3. Are the treatment methods within the scope of general practice and in keeping with the standard of care?
4. Are the outcome measures clinically important?
5. Is the follow-up greater than 80%?
6. Do the results and data support the conclusion?

The strength of different methodology and study designs in order of importance:

1. Randomized, double-blind, controlled trials
2. Quasi-randomized controlled trials
3. Nonrandomized controlled trials
4. Cohort studies with appropriately matched controls
5. Retrospective trials
6. Case reports

The ENT examination

Equipment

A full otolaryngologic examination requires certain instruments as well some specialized equipment.

Basic equipment
- A light source—a portable headlight that runs off batteries or a head mirror and halogen light source off the back of the examination chair are the standard.
- Wooden tongue depressors.
- Nasal speculum.
- An otoscope with several-sized specula.
- Ear curette for cerumen removal.
- Pneumatic attachment for the otoscope.
- Tuning fork 512 Hz.
- Angled dental mirror for evaluation of the larynx and nasopharynx.

Specialized equipment
- Anesthetic spray such as 4% lidocaine or pontocaine.
- A flexible laryngopharyngoscope with light source.
- Rigid nasal endoscope.
- Aqueous lubricating gel for the scopes.
- Suction equipment with several-size nasal and otologic suctions.
- Microalligators and forceps.

Emergency equipment
- Nasal bayonet forceps.
- Vaseline strip gauze.
- Large nasal tampons (Merocel).
- Gelfoam.
- Silver nitrate sticks.
- Foley catheter with 30 cc balloon.

Basic requirements
How to master use of a head mirror
The principle of the head mirror is that a light source is reflected from the mirror onto the patient. The mirror is concave and the light is focused to a point approximately one arm's length from the examiner. Also, it has a hole through which the examiner can look, also allowing binocular vision. Correct positioning of the examiner and the light source is important. Ensure that the light source is placed approximately level with the patient's left ear. You must sit opposite the patient with the light shining directly at your mirror. Place the mirror over the right eye, close the left eye, and adjust the mirror so that you can look through the hole directly at the patient's nose. Now adjust the light and mirror until the maximum amount of light is reflected onto the patient. When the left eye is opened, you should have binocular vision and reflected light shining to the patient's nose. The focal length of the mirror is approximately 2 feet. This means that the reflected light will be brightest and sharpest when the examiner and patient are this distance apart.

Examination of the ear

▶ Know your otoscope

The otoscope should be held like a pen with the little finger extended to touch the patient's cheek. This positioning enables an early warning of head turning, particularly in children. The right hand holds the otoscope for the right ear examination and vice versa; see Fig. 2.1.

Routine examination

- Ask the patient which is their better hearing ear and start by examining this ear.
- Check with the patient that their ear is not sore to touch.
- Examine the pinna and look for preauricular abnormalities.
- Examine for postauricular and endaural scars (see Fig. 2.2).
- Straighten the external auditory canal (EAC) by pulling the pinna up and backwards (if you are examining a baby, pull backward only).
- Examine the EAC skin and document any changes using an otoscope.
- Systematically examine the tympanic membrane.
- Visualize the handle of the malleus and follow it up to the lateral process. Then you will not miss the superior part of the drum. You may need to kneel down to get the correct angle.
- Perform a pneumatic otoscopy. It will be more accurate if you have a soft-tipped speculum that can occlude the EAC (see Fig. 2.3).
- Repeat with the pathological ear.
- Perform tuning-fork tests (see Chapter 2, p. 16).
- Perform free-field test of hearing (see Chapter 2, p. 20).
- Check facial nerve function—ask the patient to smile and close their eyes while you look for facial weakness.
- Perform cranial nerve examination (see Chapter 2, p. 34).
- Visualize the eustachian tube orifice or torus tubarius with a dental mirror or endoscope. This is especially important when examining an adult with a unilateral middle ear infection.
- Perform indirect laryngoscopy (see Chapter 2, p. 26). Visualize the larynx and hypopharynx with a dental mirror. This can be done on most individuals who can control their gag reflex.

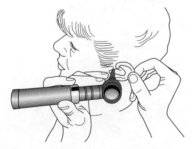

Fig. 2.1 How to hold the otoscope.

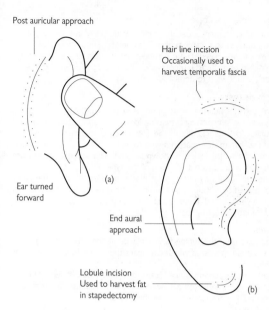

Post auricular approach

Ear turned forward

(a)

Hair line incision
Occasionally used to
harvest temporalis fascia

End aural
approach

Lobule incision
Used to harvest fat
in stapedectomy

(b)

Fig. 2.2 Common ear incisions.

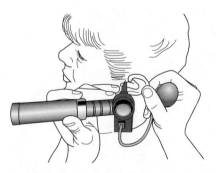

Fig. 2.3 Performance of pneumatic otoscopy.

Using an otoendoscope

The use of this instrument is becoming more widespread in Otolaryngology. It is often attached to a camera and TV monitor. The patient may enjoy seeing their ear on screen, and it can help when explaining ear pathology or surgery. No anesthetic is necessary. The end can fog up, so use an anti-fog or alcohol wipe to demist (see Fig. 2.4).

Tuning fork tests

These are tests of hearing most often used to differentiate between a conductive and a sensorineural hearing loss. They should be performed with a tuning fork of 512 Hz. If the frequency is lower, vibrations are produced that can mislead patients who think this is an auditory stimulus.

The ends of a tuning fork are known as *tynes*. The loudest sound from the tuning fork is produced at the end of the tyne.

Start the tuning fork by hitting your elbow or knee. Plucking the tynes produces less efficient sound, and hitting a table or desk edge produces overtones. Weber's and Rinne's test's are performed together to help identify the type of hearing loss.

Weber's test

In this test (Fig. 2.5), the tuning fork is placed at the top of the patient's head. The patient then says which ear hears the sound loudest, or if it is in the middle.

In normal hearing, sound is not localized to either ear. In sensorineural hearing loss, the non-affected ear hears the sound loudest. In conductive loss the sound is heard loudest in the affected ear.

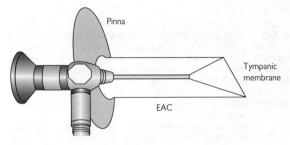

Fig. 2.4 Inserting the otoendoscope.

Pinna

Tympanic membrane

EAC

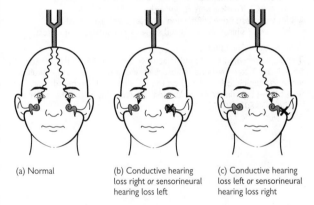

(a) Normal

(b) Conductive hearing loss right *or* sensorineural hearing loss left

(c) Conductive hearing loss left *or* sensorineural hearing loss right

Fig. 2.5 Diagram of Weber's tests.

Rinne's test

This test (Fig. 2.6) is used to compare air conduction with bone conduction. The activated tuning fork is placed behind the patient's ear, against the mastoid process. The patient is asked to say when they stop hearing the stimulus. The tuning fork is then moved to a position 2 cm away from the EAC and held with the tips of the tynes level and in line with the ear canal. The patient is then asked if they can hear the sound.

This test can be modified by moving the tuning fork from the mastoid to the EAC before the sound has diminished. The patient is then asked which is the louder sound.

The test results can be confusing, because a pathological test result is called a negative test! This is contrary to almost all other tests in medicine, where a positive result is an abnormal result and a negative result is normal. Often a description of the findings is used instead.

- **Positive test**: air conduction is better than bone conduction
  (AC > BC). This is a normal finding.
- **Negative test**: bone conduction is better than air conduction
  (BC > AC). This is abnormal and suggests conductive hearing loss.

False negative Rinne's test

This happens when the sound is actually being heard by the other ear. Sound conducted by bone is absorbed and travels across the skull, so when the tuning fork is placed on the left side it will be heard almost as well by the right inner ear as the left. To stop this effect, the other ear can be masked.

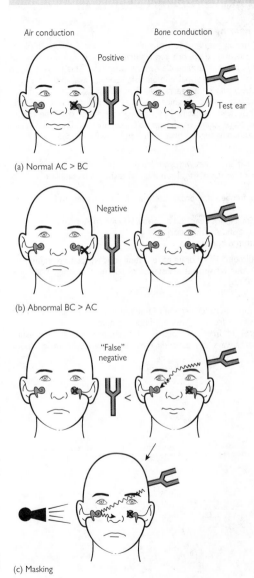

(a) Normal AC > BC

(b) Abnormal BC > AC

(c) Masking

Fig. 2.6 Diagram of Rinne's tests.

Free-field hearing tests

Patients will usually require a formal audiogram for most chronic otologic conditions. However, there are some situations when you may need to make a rough guess at a patient's hearing threshold. This might happen because there are no formal audiometric facilities available, or if you suspect a patient may be exaggerating a hearing loss.

During this test, your own voice is used as a sound stimulus, while the patient's non-test ear is masked by rubbing your finger over the tragus. This produces some sound, which helps to "mask" that ear. Practice is essential, as the positioning for this procedure can be awkward; see Fig. 2.7.

Procedure

- Shield the patient's eyes with your hand.
- With your other hand, tragal rub the non-test earn to simulate masking.
- Whisper a number at approximately 60 cm or arm's length from the test ear.
- If the patient cannot hear, use a normal-volume spoken voice, followed by a shout if necessary.
- Repeat with the opposite ear.

Patients should be 50% accurate at repeating your words to pass the test. If they hear your whisper at a distance of 60 cm, then their hearing is better than 30 dB.

▶ Examining tip

You can perform a cruder version of this test in a covert manner. When the patient sits in front of you, a whispered question as you hold the patient's notes in front of your mouth can produce an interesting response, not always corresponding to the patient's seemingly poor audiogram!

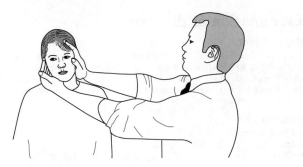

Fig. 2.7 Positioning for free-field testing.

Examination of the nose

Basic position

The patient should be sitting in a swivel chair opposite the seated examiner. It is useful to have the patient's chair slightly higher than the examiner's chair. A good light source is essential: use either a bull light positioned over the patient's left shoulder reflected onto the nose via a head mirror or a headlight. Systematically begin the exam from external to internal.

External nose

- Check for scars.
- Look at the skin type and thickness.
- Observe and palpate the nasal bones, upper lateral, and lower lateral cartilages.
- Look for symmetry and abnormal seating of the cartilages with the patient in the right and left lateral position and straight on.
- Tilt the head back to view the columella and alar cartilages in a similar way.

Internal nose

- Check the patency of each nasal airway.
- Occlude one nostril with a thumb and then ask the patient to sniff in through the nose.
- Repeat on the opposite side.
- With children a dental mirror held under the nose will show exhaled air; if there is a blockage, it will not steam up.
- Perform Cottle's test. If there is obstruction at the nasal valve, this test will improve airflow (see Fig. 2.8).
- Inspect the nose internally using the nasal speculum. An otoscope with a large speculum can be used for children. The nasal speculum is held with the dominant hand and should be inserted into the nose vertically but then rotated so that the prongs of the speculum exert pressure inferiorly and superiorly. Avoid placing pressure on the nasal septum, as this area is highly sensitive and bleeds easily.
- Assess the straightness and integrity of the septum.
- Assess the size and appearance of the turbinates.
- Note the mucosal appearance and look for the presence of polyps.
- Use the endoscope to assess the posterior part of the nose.

Nasopharyngeal examination (indirect nasopharyngoscopy)

See Fig. 2.9.
- Inspect the posterior choana and nasopharynx with an endoscope or a mirror.
- Anesthetize the oropharynx.
- Hold a tongue depressor in the right hand and use it to depress the patient's tongue.
- In the other hand, use a small mirror and run it along the top of the tongue depressor to enter the oropharynx behind the soft palate.
- The reflected light should illuminate the nasopharynx to visualize the posterior choana and the ends of the inferior turbinates. Any adenoid tissue will also be seen.

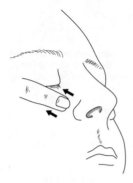

Fig. 2.8 Diagram of Cottle's test (Lift the skin upward and laterally to see if there is an improvement in nasal patency.)

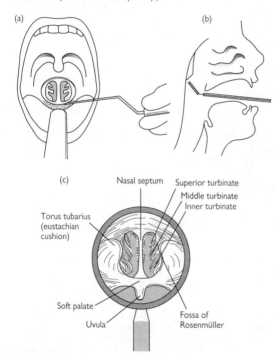

Fig. 2.9 Diagram of visualization of nasopharynx.

Rigid nasal endoscopy

Procedure

Nasal endoscopy is commonly used to evaluate the nasal cavity and nasopharynx and is especially valuable for the evaluation of nasal polyps and abnormal anatomy. The endoscope is often used for suctioning, debridement, and instrumentation of the nasal cavity.

- Before starting, warn the patient that the nasal spray tastes dreadful, that their throat will be numb, and that food or drink should not be consumed for an hour.
- Prepare the patient's nose with lidocaine or cophenylcaine spray, usually two sprays to each nostril. The anesthetic and vasoconstrictive effect of the spray takes several minutes to work, so it is essential to wait before starting the procedure.
- A standard nasal endoscope is 4 mm in diameter and angled either 0° or 30°. A 2.7 mm scope can be helpful in a narrow nose.
- Use the standard three-pass technique as shown in Fig. 2.10. Fig. 2.11 shows the differing views of the nasal anatomy on the three passes.

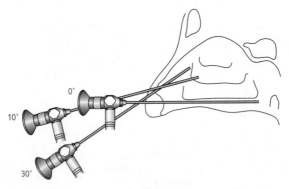

Fig. 2.10 Diagram of three-pass technique.

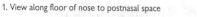

1. View along floor of nose to postnasal space

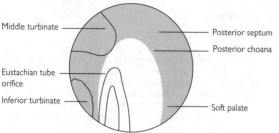

Middle turbinate ——————

Posterior septum

Posterior choana

Eustachian tube orifice

Inferior turbinate ——————

Soft palate

2. View into middle meatus

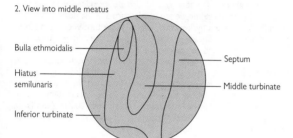

Bulla ethmoidalis ——————

Hiatus semilunaris ——————

Inferior turbinate ——————

Septum

Middle turbinate

3. View into frontal recess

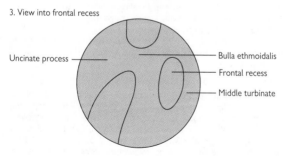

Uncinate process ——————

Bulla ethmoidalis

Frontal recess

Middle turbinate

Fig. 2.11 Views on endoscopy seen during passes in right nasal cavity.

Examination of the mouth, larynx, and pharynx

Examination of the oral cavity

A good light source is essential. Ask the patient to remove all dentures to avoid missing important pathology. Ask the patient to open their mouth wide; limitation of jaw opening (trismus) may occur as a result of acute inflammation or tumor infiltration of the muscles of mastication. Trismus is graded on the basis of interincisor distance. A normal interincisor distance is greater than 3.5 cm. In an orderly way, inspect the different components of the tongue. Pay particular attention to the lateral edges of the tongue, especially posteriorly. It may be necessary to use the tongue depressor to push the tongue medially to adequately examine this area. Any abnormality seen should also be examined with a gloved finger, since tumors of the tongue are usually hard and the depth of invasion can be difficult to assess by inspection alone. Now turn your attention to the floor of the mouth, the lower teeth, and gums. Use a tongue depressor to distract the cheek and to look at the parotid duct opening (Stenson's duct), opposite the second upper molar tooth. Inspect both hard and soft palate. Inspect in turn each of the tonsils, as well as the posterior pharyngeal wall. Test the movements of the palate by asking the patient to say "aahh" and the integrity of the hypoglossal nerve by asking them to stick out their tongue. The best way to assess the submandibular gland is via bimanual palpation with one hand placed on the neck and a gloved finger of the other in the floor of the mouth.

Examination of the larynx and pharynx

A lot of information can be gained by simply listening to the patient's voice. A weak, breathy voice with a poor cough may suggest vocal cord palsy. A harsh, hoarse voice is suggestive of a vocal cord lesion. With experience one can also recognize the characteristic voice of vocal cord nodules and Reinke's edema; however, the definitive diagnosis depends on inspection of the vocal cords.

How to perform indirect laryngoscopy

Positioning of the patient is very important; the patient should be placed leaning slightly forward with the head slightly extended. An appropriately sized laryngeal mirror should be selected that is large enough to give a good view but small enough to be placed comfortably at the back of the mouth. Spraying the oral cavity with a topical anesthetic may help. The mirrored surface should be gently warmed using warm beads, hot water, or an electrical mirror warmer. Have the patient go into a sniffing position with their back straight and slightly inclined towards you. The chin should be extended slightly forward, Position the light directly into the oropharynx. Have the patient open their mouth and pull the tongue forward with a gauze pad. Insert the dental mirror through the mouth with it angled inferiorly, trying to avoid the base of tongue and the lateral tonsillar pillars. Lift the soft palate posteriorly, and the hypopharynx and larynx should come into view (see Fig. 2.12). Ask the patient to concentrate on their breathing; sometimes asking them to pant helps them to focus further and also improves your view. Ask the patient to say "eeee" and note the movements of the vocal cords.

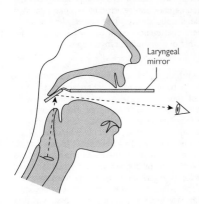

Laryngeal
mirror

Fig. 2.12 Indirect laryngoscopy.

Flexible laryngoscopy

Flexible direct laryngoscopy is a very important component of examining the upper aerodigestive tract. This is easy to perform in the outpatient clinic, usually with the aid of some topical decongestant and anesthetic. Unlike rigid telescopes, which have sets of lens arranged longitudinally, the flexible laryngoscope (sometimes also referred to as a nasopharyngoscope) is traditionally a fiber-optic device. The newer, flexible endoscopes have a digital camera chip embedded in the distal tip, and offer greater image quality than that of fiber-optic laryngoscopes.

Technique

The flexible scope is passed through the nose, giving the opportunity to inspect the middle and inferior turbinates, nasal septum, and osteomeatal complex. The presence of mucopus, nasal septal deviation, vascular ectasias. and abnormal nasal anatomy should be noted. The endoscope is then advanced to the nasopharynx where the eustachian tube orifices, fossa of Rosenmuller, and adenoids can be seen. The function of the velopharyngeal complex can be seen by asking the patient to say "kaa kaa kaa." This will raise the palate to form a complete seal around the nasopharynx. The presence of secretions or bubbles in the nasopharynx with this maneuver suggests velopharyngeal insufficiency. By advancing past the superior aspect of the soft palate the endoscopist can see the tongue base, lingual tonsils, vallecula, laryngeal inlet, and pyriform fossa. Visualization of these areas can be improved by asking the patient to stick out their tongue and also performing a Valsalva maneuver while the examiner pinches the patient's nose to prevent air escape. Special care should be made to evaluate the pyriform fossa, which is an area difficult to assess and can hide a malignancy.

Movements of the vocal cords can be assessed by asking the patient to speak. Connected speech function and vocal fold movement are evaluated and the presence of hyperfunction checked (does the false vocal fold overshadow the true vocal folds during speech?). Evidence of tremor or dystonia should also be noted. Any mucosal abnormalities should be carefully examined and documented. The patient should be asked to cough and clear their throat and to swallow, to assess these vegetative tasks.

Special tests such as functional endoscopic evaluation of swallowing (FEES) and the Muller maneuver for obstructive sleep apnea can also be performed with the flexible laryngoscope.

Stroboscopy

Fine movements of the vocal cords and mucosal wave require strobo-scopic examination. A microphone is placed on the neck and the fre-quency of vocal cord vibration is matched to the frequency of a strobe light flashing. The resulting image shown is a slow-motion, moving image of the vocal cords. The *mucosal wave* is the undulation of the superficial layers of the vocal cord, which produces sound and pitch through vibration. The *vocal cords* are folds of tissue composed of the muscle, ligament, soft tissue, and epithelium. The vocal cords are the principal sound generator for phonation. The image is captured from a 60° or 70° rigid telescope inserted into the mouth. Flexible distal-chip digital endoscopes are capable of rendering detailed images of the mucosal wave and can also be used for stroboscopic evaluation.

Technique

Insertion of the rigid telescope is poorly tolerated in patients with a hypersensitive gag reflex, and the technique requires practice to master. The patient sits upright and leans slightly forward with the chin extended in a "sniffing" position. The tongue is extended and gently grasped and retracted forward. The telescope is inserted into the oral cavity carefully; the anterior tonsillar pillars and base of tongue should be avoided. The angulation of the telescope is designed so that the glottis is visualized as the tip of the scope is in the oropharynx. The patient is asked to sustain a long |a|, at several different pitches and the mucosal wave is evaluated. Vocal fold nodules, scar, sulcus, varices, hemorrhages, and polyps are often evaluated with stroboscopy. See Fig. 2.13 for an image of the vocal folds seen with a rigid endoscope.

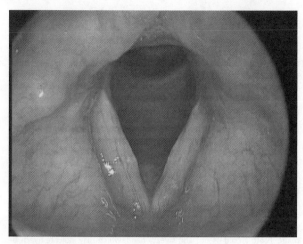

Fig. 2.13 View of the larynx through the laryngoscope.

Examination of the neck

Start by inspecting the neck from the front. Look for any scars, masses, deformity, or asymmetry that may be visible. Ask the patient to swallow and pay particular attention to the lower central neck, looking for a thyroid mass, which should rise on swallowing. Again, a systematic examination will ensure that no area is missed. See Fig. 2.14, which illustrates a suggested method of examination.

Examination of a neck mass

If you do find a mass or abnormality, ensure that you can adequately describe it and how it is related to the anatomy of the neck—i.e., site, size, consistency, surface, mobility; is it single or pulsatile? The position of a neck mass will give clues as to the likely cause. Fig. 2.15 gives a list of the common differential diagnoses, depending on the site of the mass.

Examination of the thyroid

Thyroid masses are common and often appear in exams. Because of the systemic nature of thyroid disorders, some additional points are important to demonstrate. An overview of the patient's appearance should be made. Note a cold or hot and sweaty hand, which may indicate hypo- or hyperthyroidism, respectively; similarly, look at the skin and hair quality. Look for loss of the outer third of the eyebrow, which may occur in hypothyroid function. Look at the neck from the front and ask the patient to swallow, noting any thyroid masses that will rise during swallowing.

Ask the patient to cough, listening for a weak cough and breathy voice, which may occur in a recurrent laryngeal nerve palsy due to malignant infiltration of the nerve. Now move behind the patient and feel the midline from the chin to the sternal notch. Feel for any midline lumps, especially thyroglossal cysts, which will elevate on protrusion of the tongue, distinguishing them from the thyroid isthmus. Remember that the normal thyroid gland is soft and difficult to distinguish from surrounding soft tissue. Feel each of the lobes in turn as well as the isthmus, asking the patient to swallow once more and checking if any palpable mass rises during swallowing.

Examination of salivary glands

Palpation of the parotid gland should be included in the routine examination of the neck. Remember that most parotid masses are found just behind the angle of the mandible and that the tail of the parotid gland can extend down into the neck as far as the hyoid. Tumors of the deep lobe of the parotid may present as a mass arising in the mouth and pushing the tonsil medially. Examination of the parotid gland includes testing the function of the facial nerve and visualization and palpation of the duct.

Submandibular gland masses are best felt via bimanual palpation. Remember to also inspect and palpate the length of the submandibular duct as it runs along the floor of the mouth and opens at a punctum next to the frenulum of the tongue.

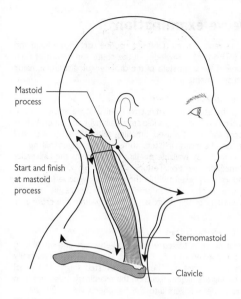

Fig. 2.14 Systematic examination of the neck.

Mastoid process

Start and finish at mastoid process

Sternomastoid

Clavicle

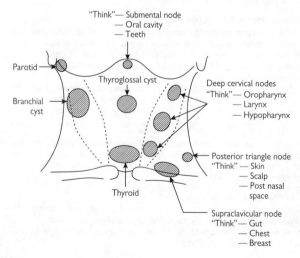

"Think"— Submental node
— Oral cavity
— Teeth

Parotid

Thyroglossal cyst

Branchial cyst

Deep cervical nodes
"Think"— Oropharynx
— Larynx
— Hypopharynx

Posterior triangle node
"Think"— Skin
— Scalp
— Post nasal space

Thyroid

Supraclavicular node
"Think"— Gut
— Chest
— Breast

Fig. 2.15 Diagram of neck masses by position and likely diagnosis.

Cranial nerve examination

Examination of the cranial nerves (CN) is a routine part of the head and neck examination. Thorough knowledge of the route and nature of each cranial nerve is one of the basic skills of the otolaryngologist and a major tool in the clinical armamentarium.

Cranial nerve I—olfactory nerve

Olfaction is tested by asking the patient to smell and describe a scent. Commonly used are cloves or spices kept in an air-tight container. Wipes with a lemon scent can also be used. Smelling salts and alcohol should not be used, as the chemicals' irritants stimulate the trigeminal nerve. There are also commercially available smelling tests such as the University of Pennsylvania Smell Identification Test.

The sensory fibers are present within the olfactory groove just below the cribriform plate. Problems with smell can be the result of nasal obstruction or disorders of the neurosensory cells within the groove or the frontal lobe.

Cranial nerve II—optic nerve

The second cranial nerve is tested with a Snellen chart and visual-field testing. The patient is asked to hold the chart at arm's length (generally 20 cm) and to recite each letter. The eyes are tested singly. The visual field is tested by having the patient fixate on the examiner's nose and then introducing the examiner's fingers into the peripheral vision. By keeping the hands an equal distance apart, the examiner can compare the patient's visual field with his or her own.

Cranial nerve III—oculomotor nerve

The oculomotor nerve innervates most of the extraocular muscles—the superior rectus, medial rectus, inferior rectus, and inferior oblique as well as the levator palpebrae superioris. The examination is composed of having the patient track the finger of the examiner into all four quadrants of the visual field.

CNIII also has a parasympathetic function, which arises from the Edinger–Westphal nucleus. The fibers carry signal to the ciliary muscles and sphincter pupillae muscles, which regulate papillary dilation.

Cranial nerve IV—trochlear nerve

The trochlear nerve innervates the superior oblique muscle. Isolated dysfunction of CNIV can be subtle. The paralysis results in outward rotation of the eye and weakness of downward gaze. Patients commonly complain of difficulty going down stairs.

Cranial nerve V—trigeminal nerve

The trigeminal nerve has motor and sensory functions and is traditionally divided into three major divisions. The trigeminal ganglion sits in Meckel's cave, which is in the floor of the middle cranial fossa. Testing is performed with a cotton-tipped applicator.

- V3: The **mandibular division** of the trigeminal nerve, or V3, provides sensation into the lower face as well as the mouth. The sensory nerves include the buccal, auriculotemporal, lingual, inferior alveolar, and meningeal branches. The mandibular branch also has motor function, providing innervation to the muscles of mastication—the tensor tympani, tensor veli palatini, mylohyoid, and anterior belly of the digastric muscles.
- V2: The **maxillary division** of the trigeminal nerve, or V2, provides sensation to the mid-face. The sensory branches are carried by the zygomatic, infraorbital, ptyerygopalatine, and meningeal nerves.
- V1: The **ophthalmic division** is primarily sensory. The signal is carried by the lacimal, frontal, nasopharyngeal, and meningeal nerves. Parasympathetic fibers originating from the facial nerve, CNVII, join the lacrimal nerve.

The *corneal reflex* tests the reflex arc between CNV and CNVII and may be a subtle finding associated with cerebellopontine angle (CPA) lesions. Use a cotton ball to stimulate the lateral conjunctiva to reflexively close the eye.

Cranial nerve VI—abducens nerve

The abducens nerve innervates the lateral rectus muscle. Dysfunction of CNVI results in difficulty rotating the globe medially, leading to double vision, or diplopia.

Cranial nerve VII—facial nerve

Anatomy

The facial nerve has motor, sensory, including special sensory of taste, and parasympathetic functions. The convergence and divergence of the various fibers from one nerve to branches of other cranial nerves can produce significant confusion. It is important to study the path and function of this nerve carefully.

The facial-nerve anatomy is often classified by its position in relationship to the temporal bone; it is divided into an intracranial component, intratemporal segment (which is further divided into a meatal, labyrinthine, tympanic [horizontal], and mastoid [vertical] component), and extratemporal segments.

The *nervus intermedius* provides the parasympathiec and sensory fibers of the facial nerve. The motor nucleus joins the nervus intermediasis within the CPA to form the common facial nerve.

The nerve enters the internal auditory meatus and enters the temporal bone. The nerve makes its first turn, or *first genu*, at the *geniculate ganglion*, which houses sensory neurons. The *greater superficial petrosal nerve* is the first branch off the facial nerve and carries preganglionic parasympathetic fibers to the lacrimal gland.

After the first genu, the tympanic segment of the nerve enters the middle ear and courses between the oval window and stapes. The bony covering in the tympanic segment may be dehiscent, and this is an area of vulnerability for the nerve during ear infections and otologic surgery.

The nerve then makes a second turn, or *second genu*, and enters a vertical pathway down the mastoid portion of the temporal bone. The *stapedial nerve*, which innervates the stapedius muscle as well as the *chorda tympani*, which carries parasympathetic fibers and special sensory of taste fibers (provides taste to the anterior two thirds of the tongue) to the lingual nerve (of CNV), branches off at this region.

The nerve then leaves the temporal bone via the *stylomastoid foramen*.

The facial nerve provides innervation to the muscles of facial expression, the *stylohyoid nerve*, the nerve to the *posterior digastric*, and *postauricular nerve*. The innervation to the facial muscles is carried out via the five divisions of the main motor trunk, called the *Pes anserinus*: the *temporal, zygomatic, buccal, mandibular,* and *cervical branches*.

Cranial nerve VII—facial nerve

Functional testing

The facial nerve has motor and sensory function, provides special sensory of taste, and has parasympathetic function.

Motor function is tested by asking the patient to smile, grimace, wrinkle the nose, close the eye, and raise the eyebrows. The *House–Brackman scale* (Table 2.1) is used to describe the severity of paralysis. Also look for tics, spasms, and synkinesis.

Dysfunction at the brainstem or central nervous system (CNS) level can be differentiated from peripheral nerve dysfunction by the movement at the forehead. Centrally, there is bilateral innervation of the motor nerve nucleus; therefore, CNS disorders producing facial paralysis will have intact forehead movement. Peripheral disorders will result in paralysis of the forehead as well.

Lacrimal function and tear production can be assessed with *Shirmer's test*, which involves placing a filter paper strip at the corner of the lateral canthus.

The sensory component of the facial nerve can be assessed by sensory testing of the concha of the external ear, the postauricular skin, and wall of the external auditory canal (*Hitselberger sign*).

Taste is often difficult to test because of bilateral innervation of the chorda tympani, the sensory component provided by CNV and CNIX, and the substantial role of smell in taste cues. Patients with chorda tympani dysfunction often complain of a metallic taste or alterations in taste.

Patients may also complain of hypersensitivity to loud noises or hyperacusis, because the stapedius muscle has a role in dampening sounds. The stapedial reflex may be tested on the audiogram; however, a significant percentage of the normal population lack the stapedial reflex on testing.

Facial nerve dysfunction with diplopia suggests an injury at the brainstem as the facial nerve motor fibers loop around the abducens motor nucleus.

Ancillary testing such as electromyography (EMG) or electroneuronography (ENoG) may be useful in the setting of facial nerve paralysis.

Table 2.1 House–Brackman facial nerve grading scale

I	Normal
II	Normal tone and symmetry at rest
	Slight weakness and asymmetry with maximal effort
III	Normal tone and symmetry at rest
	Obvious weakness and asymmetry with effort
	Mild synkinesis or hemifacial spasms
	Good eye closure
IV	Normal tone and symmetry at rest
	Disfiguring asymmetry and weakness
	Incomplete eye closure
V	Poor tone and asymmetric at rest
	Very slight movement with maximal effort
VI	No motion

House JW and Brackmann DE. (1985). Facial nerve grading system. *Otolaryngol Head Neck Surg* **193**:146.

Cranial nerve VIII—vestibulocochlear nerve

The vestibulococlear nerve is a special sensory nerve that carries auditory and vestibular information from the cochlea, utricle, saccule, and semicircular canals.

The hearing test may be performed with tuning forks, free-field testing, and formal audiometry. The vestibular function may be assessed by testing the extraocular nerves for nystagmus, gait and balance testing, Romberg testing and Unterberger stepping test, and finger-to-nose testing.

Romberg test Have the patient stand straight with eyes closed and feet parallel and slightly less than shoulder length apart. Stand at the side and be prepared to stabilize the patient in case of fall. Normally, this position should be maintained for greater than 30 seconds without significant body sway.

Unterberger stepping test Have the patient march in step with eyes closed. Unilateral vestibular dysfunction will often result in the patient rotating toward the side of the lesion.

Nystagmus refers to rhythmic eye movements that occur with visual tracking. Have the patient track your finger horizontally and then vertically across the visual field. Carefully observe the pupils at rest. There is a fast twitch or jerk of the eyes followed by a slow correction. Nystagmus may by physiologic, induced (such as during caloric testing or Dix–Hallpike maneuvers), or pathologic. Pathological or *spontaneous nystagmus* is present at rest within 30° of the central visual field. Physiologic nystagmus is present at the lateral gazes. The *direction* of the nystagmus, by convention, is described by the direction of the fast phase.

Cranial nerve IX—glossopharyngeal nerve

The glossopharyngeal nerve provides special taste sensation and general sensation to the posterior one-third of the tongue, motor function to the *stylopharyngeus muscle*, parasympathetic stimulation to the parotid gland via *Jacobson's nerve*, visceral sensory signal from the carotid body and sinus, and sensory signal from the external auditory canal and medial surface of the tympanic membrane.

The motor function of CNIX is tested by watching the symmetry and movement of the soft palate. Unilateral weakness is usually seen as deviation of the uvula away from the affected side.

The sensory function of CNIX is tested by stimulating the back of the tongue and soft palate. A decreased gag reflex suggests dysfunction.

Throat pain and ear pain often occur together because of the common nerve fibers.

CNIX often has dysfunction with other cranial nerves that exit the skull from the jugular foramen. The associated cranial neuropathies are referred to as *jugular foramen syndrome* and involve dysfunction on CNIX, X, XI, and XII.

Cranial nerve X—vagus nerve

The vagus nerve has motor, somatic sensory, and visceral sensory functions. CNX is widely dispersed throughout the body and has major regulatory functions outside the head and neck involving the respiratory, gastrointestinal, and cardiovascular systems.

The motor function involves innervation of the muscles of the pharynx and larynx. It also provides visceral function and innervation to the smooth muscles and glands of the pharynx, larynx, thorax, and abdomen.

The head and neck sensory component of the vagus is carried from the external ear canal and lateral tympanic membrane (via *Arnold's nerve*) as well as the pharynx and larynx.

Like CNIX, the motor function of CNX is tested by watching the symmetry and movement of the soft palate. Unilateral weakness is usually seen as deviation of the uvula away from the affected side.

The *recurrent laryngeal nerve* and *superior laryngeal nerve* are branches from the vagus that innervate the larynx. Evaluation of vocal fold movement for evidence of paralysis is performed with indirect or direct laryngoscopy. The flexible laryngoscope can also be used to gently touch the arytenoids and aryepiglottic (AE) folds to evaluate the sensory function of the vagus via the superior laryngeal nerve.

Cranial nerve XI—spinal accessory nerve

The spinal accessory nerve is a pure motor nerve that provides innervation to the sternocleidomastoid and the trapezius muscles. Weakness of these muscles is tested by firmly clasping the shoulder and asking the patient to shrug against resistance.

Dysfunction of CNXI is most commonly seen after neck surgery and it is often removed during cancer resection.

Cranial nerve XII—hypoglossal nerve

The hypoglossal nerve is another pure motor nerve that innervates the tongue. The nerve is tested by asking the patient to protrude the tongue fully and moving it from side to side and vertically. A unilateral lesion of the hypoglossal nerve results in the tongue protruding toward the side of dysfunction.

Recommended reading

Wilson-Pauwells L, Akesson E, Stewart P, and Spacy S. (2005). *Cranial Nerves in Health and Disease*, 2nd ed. New York: BC Decker.

Common methods of presentation

Hoarse voice

History	Examination		Diagnosis	Page no.
Lasted less than 2 weeks + fever + a sore throat + URTI symptoms	→ Diffusely inflamed larynx		Acute laryngitis	170
Lasting more than 3 weeks	→ Vocal cord lesion	Unilateral	Vocal polyp Vocal granuloma Papilloma	180 180 181
		Bilateral	Papillomata Vocal nodules Sulcus and scarring Thin atrophic vocal folds presbylarynges	181
Lasted more than 3 weeks Constant Progressive Patient is a smoker —dysphagia —pain —otalgia —a neck lump	→ Vocal cord lesion	Unilateral	Laryngeal cancer	174
		Bilateral	Reinkes edema	171

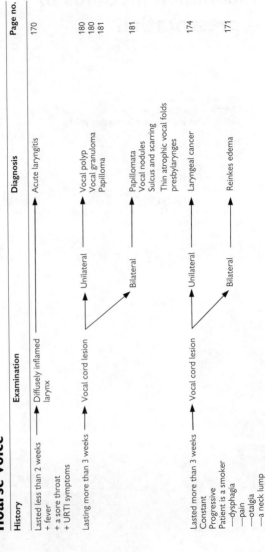

Variable with history of ———▶ Restricted vocal fold ———▶ Vocal fold immobility
surgery, head and neck or   movement   Neurological paralysis or paresis—
thoracic malignancy, or   recurrent laryngeal nerve, vagus nerve,
trauma   or brainstem lesion
                                                        Mechanical immobility—arytenoids subluxa-
                                                        tion, dislocation, or arthritis.
                                                        Posterior glottic scarring and stenosis

Variable
Strained or raspy voice ———▶ No vocal cord lesion   181

                                             Muscle tension dysphonia
                                             Spasmodic dysphonia
                                             Functional dysphonia
                                             Malingering
                                             hypothyroidism

Epistaxis (nosebleed)

History	Examination	Diagnosis/treatment	Page no.
Trauma or injury has occured	Anterior bleed → Blood vessels on Little's area	First line • First aid • Nasal cautery • Nasal packing	412 392 394
Hypertension			
Anticoagulation		Second line	
Aspirin use		• Bilateral posterior packing	
Bleeding tendency		• Interventional angiogram and occlusion	
Hemophilia	Posterior bleed → Blood in the posterior nasal cavity	• Ligation of internal maxillary artery	
Leukemia/lymphoma			
Platelet dysfunction			
Cocaine abuse			
Multiple telangectasias		Osler–Weber–Rendu syndrome or hereditary hemorrhagic telangiectasias (HHT)	412
+ nasal obstruction + serosanguinous discharge + facial swelling + proptosis + facial paresthesia + a neck lump		Sinonasal tumors Abscess and infection (fungal, syphilis, TB) Granulomatous disease	324
Adolescent boys	Nasal mass/polyp	Angiofibroma	

Dysphagia (swallowing difficulty)

History	Examination	Diagnosis	Page no.
Constant	Neck mass	Carcinoma	200
Progressive	Endoscopy—lesion seen		196
Solids worse than liquids			197
Pain			
Otalgia	Endoscopy—pooling of saliva	Post-cricoid web	
Neck lump		Achalasia	
		Stenosis/stricture	
		Esophageal web	
		Diffuse posterior osteophytes	
		Infectious esophagitis—fungal, viral, or bacterial	
Constant	Pouch or diverticulum on barium swallow	Pharyngeal pouch or Zenker's diverticulum	198
Progressive			
Regurgitation	Fistula or connection with trachea on barium swallow	Tracheoesophageal fistula	
Halitosis		Laryngeal cleft	
Aspiration			
Cough			
Pneumonias			

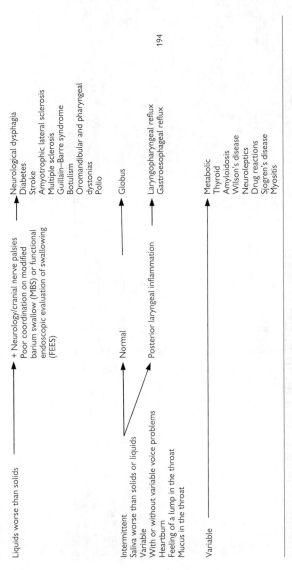

Liquids worse than solids ⟶ + Neurology/cranial nerve palsies
Poor coordination on modified
barium swallow (MBS) or functional
endoscopic evaluation of swallowing
(FEES) ⟶ Neurological dysphagia
Diabetes
Stroke
Amyotrophic lateral sclerosis
Multiple sclerosis
Guillain–Barre syndrome
Botulism
Oromandibular and pharyngeal
dystonias
Polio

Intermittent
Saliva worse than solids or liquids
Variable ⟶ Normal ⟶ Globus

With or without variable voice problems
Heartburn ⟶ Posterior laryngeal inflammation ⟶ Laryngopharyngeal reflux
Gastroesophageal reflux   194
Feeling of a lump in the throat
Mucus in the throat

Variable ⟶ Metabolic
Thyroid
Amyloidosis
Wilson's disease
Neuroleptics
Drug reactions
Sjogren's disease
Myositis

Globus (a feeling of a lump in the throat)

History	Examination	Diagnosis	Page no.
Constant	Lesion seen on examination	Carcinoma of pharynx	193
Same site	Neck mass	Carcinoma of esophagus	
Worse with solids			
Unilateral			
pain			
otalgia			
neck mass			
hoarse voice			
Smoking history			
Foreign body ingestion	Foreign body on endoscopy	Foreign body ingestion	
Constant and same side			
Fever and pain			
Variable site	Examination normal	Globus	
Comes and goes			
Worse with saliva	Posterior laryngeal edema	Laryngopharyngeal reflux	
Central in the neck			
Variable voice problems	Rhinosinusitis and seasonal allergies	Rhinogenic laryngitis	
Heart burn/reflux			

Neck mass

All of those below may apply to children, but most neck masses in children are benign and are reactive lymph nodes. Parotid masses in children are more frequently malignant than in adults.

History	Examination	Diagnosis	Page no.
Short history (weeks/months)	→ Laterally placed	Malignant lymphadenopathy	208
Lump is enlarging	Firm/hard	Head and neck primary	
Unilateral nasal obstruction	Single	Squamous cell carcinoma	
Otalgia	Immobile	Thyroid cancer—metastatic	
Sore throat		Carotid body tumor	
Patient is a smoker			
Hoarse voice			
Swallowing problems			
Weight loss	→ Multiple mobile enlarged	Malignant lymphoma	
Night sweats	lymphadenopathy	Glandular fever/toxoplasma	99
Anorexia	Rubbery	Parotitis, cat scratch disease	
Fever	Groin/axillary nodes	Tuberculosis	
Foreign travel		Kikuchis' disease	
		Granulomatous disease	
		Sarcoid	

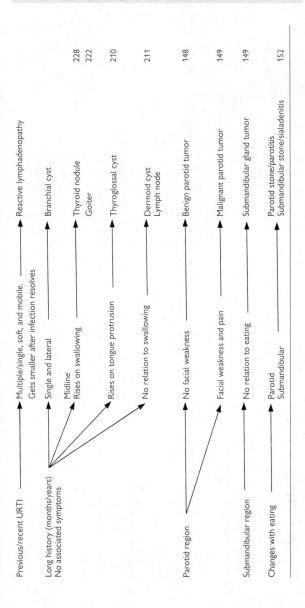

Mouth or tongue ulcer

History	Examination	Diagnosis	Page no.
Trauma or injury Poor-fitting denture Sharp tooth pain	Lateral tongue Buccal mucosa	→ Traumatic ulcer	88
Tobacco use Alcohol Betel nut chewer Progressive Pain Neck mass Otalgia	Lateral tongue Floor of mouth Tonsil Firm/hard ulcer Neck nodes	→ Malignant ulcer (SCC)	90
Normal immune function Recurrent	Multiple ulcers Tongue tip/lateral border	→ Aphthous ulcers	88
Infectious		Candida Herpes simplex Herpangina (coxsackievirus) Parvovirus Varicella Syphilus	

Drug reaction ⟶ Steven's Johnson syndrome
Erythema multiforme

Poor dental hygiene ⟶ Necrotizine ulcerative
gingival stomatitis

Associated with systemic ⟶ Systemic lupus
disorders erythromatosus
Inflammatory bowel
disease
Lichen planus
Pemphigus
Bullous pemphigus
Behcet's disease

Dietary insufficiency ⟶ Dietary/blood disorders 89

Angular stomatitis
Skin lesions

Stridor

History	Examination	Diagnosis	Page no.
Neonate			
Feeding problems	Positional	Laryngomalacia	168
Failure to thrive		Tracheomalacia	168
Abnormal cry		Vocal cord lesion/palsy	169
	Biphasic stridor	Subglottic stenosis	168
	Aspiration is prominent	Tracheoesophageal fistula	
		Laryngeal cleft	
Child			
Preceding URTI	Drooling	Croup	172
Rapid onset	Pyrexia	Epiglottitis	171
Malaise	Toxic	Deep neck abscess	
Voice muffled/changed			
Short history	Inspiratory/mixed stridor	Foreign body	185
Previously well child	Expiratory wheeze		
Short-lived coughing fit			
Adult			
Normal voice	Inspiratory stridor	Bilateral cord immobility	185
Recent surgery (thyroid/chest)		Laryngeal stenosis	
		Laryngeal granuloma	

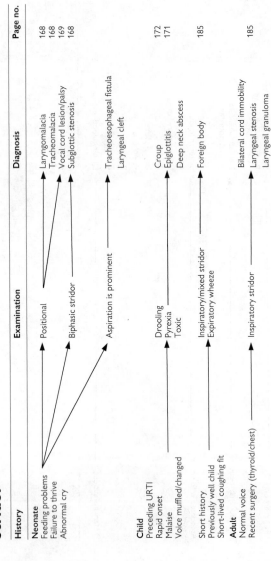

Preceding URTI
Malaise
Swallowing difficulty
Sore throat

Inspiratory stridor
Pyrexia
Drooling

→ Supraglottitis
Deep neck abscess, parapharyn-   185
geal,
retropharyngeal spaces
Angioedema
Ludwigs angina

Anxious patient

Variable inspiratory stridor
No cyanosis

→ Paradoxical vocal fold
movement laryngospasm
Laryngeal dystonia

Long-standing hoarse voice
Pain
Patient is a smoker

Inspiratory stridor
Neck mass

→ Laryngeal carcinoma   174

Facial nerve palsy

History	Examination	Diagnosis	Page no.
Recent trauma Hemotympanum	Head injury Trauma to ear canal/drum CSF from ear/nose Battle's sign (bilateral ecchymosis at mastoid process)	Fractured temporal bone	
Rapid onset Other weakness	Forehead unaffected Abnormal neurological exam	Cerebrovascular accident (CVA)	
Rapid onset Isolated weakness Otalgia	Forehead affected Vesicles in ear	Bell's palsy Ramsay Hunt syndrome	415
Gradual onset Other weakness	Abnormal neurological exam	Multiple sclerosis (MS) Motor neuron disease Guillain–Barre syndrome Lyme disease	251
Gradual onset Facial pain	Parotid mass	Parotid carcinoma	
Hearing loss Balance disturbance	Sensorineural hearing loss Ataxia	CPA tumor Acoustic neuroma (Vestibular schwannoma) Meningioma Epidermoid tumor	
Ear discharge	Conductive hearing loss	Cholesteatoma Malignant otitis externa	

Nasal obstruction

Careful examination of the nasal anatomy will reveal what is responsible for nasal obstruction. Always remember that several anatomical problems can coexist. Symptoms can vary, especially for mucosal problems, so ascertain the severity of the problem when you examine the patient's nose.

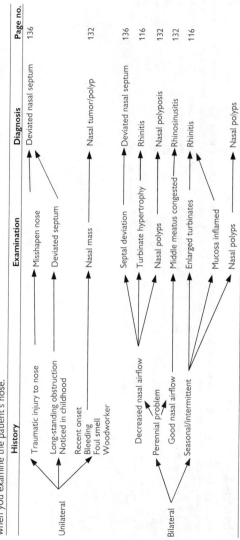

History	Examination	Diagnosis	Page no.
Unilateral			
Traumatic injury to nose	Misshapen nose	Deviated nasal septum	136
Long-standing obstruction Noticed in childhood	Deviated septum		
Recent onset Bleeding Foul smell Woodworker	Nasal mass	Nasal tumor/polyp	132
Bilateral			
Decreased nasal airflow	Septal deviation	Deviated nasal septum	136
	Turbinate hypertrophy	Rhinitis	116
Perennial problem	Nasal polyps	Nasal polyposis	132
Good nasal airflow	Middle meatus congested	Rhinosinusitis	132
Seasonal/intermittent	Enlarged turbinates	Rhinitis	116
	Mucosa inflamed		
	Nasal polyps	Nasal polyps	

Otorrhea

The timing of the onset of discharge in relation to any pain often helps with diagnosis. Otitis externa in particular can be secondary to infection spreading from the middle ear. Microsuction, or dry mopping, is often necessary to visualize the tympanic membrane. A final diagnosis is sometimes not possible until the ear has been cleaned and the local infection has been treated. It is important to visualize the ear drum after treatment in order to exclude serious pathology at the level of the tympanic membrane.

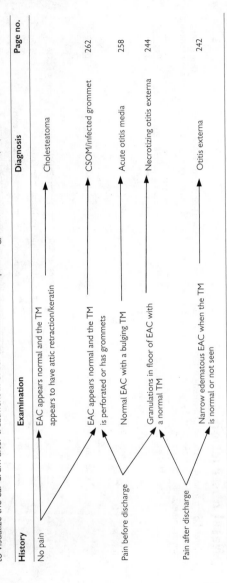

History	Examination	Diagnosis	Page no.
No pain	EAC appears normal and the TM appears to have attic retraction/keratin	Cholesteatoma	
	EAC appears normal and the TM is perforated or has grommets	CSOM/infected grommet	262
Pain before discharge	Normal EAC with a bulging TM	Acute otitis media	258
	Granulations in floor of EAC with a normal TM	Necrotizing otitis externa	244
Pain after discharge	Narrow edematous EAC when the TM is normal or not seen	Otitis externa	242

Dizziness and vertigo

The most important aspect here is the patient's history. Take great care to elicit the character of the dizziness and its time course to establish if this is dizziness or true vertigo.

History	Examination	Diagnosis	Page no.
Lasts for **seconds** Positional	Hallpike test +ve Normal pure tone averages (PTA)	BPPV	302
Lasts for **hours** Aural fullness	PTA fluctuating sensorineural loss	Meniere's disease	304
	PTA normal	Perilymphatic fistula	
Lasts for **days**		Vestibulitis or labyrinthitis	300
Single severe attack	Unterberger's test +ve	Cerebrovascular event	
variable	Normal PTA	migraine—vertebrobasilar type Multiple sclerosis AV malformation	
Constant Elderly patient	PTA normal Vestibular function tests normal	Multifactorial causes, consider: Neurodegenerative Loss of proprioception Poor vision	
Intermittent	PTA normal	Ototoxicity or vestibular toxicity (aminoglycoside) Drug related. Decompensation	292
Previous severe attack of vertigo	PTA asymmetric hearing loss Vestibular testing abnormal	CPA tumor Acoustic neuroma	

True Vertigo

Disequilibrium

Otalgia (earache)

Patients who present with otalgia can present a challenging problem. A careful history can help distinguish many conditions. Watch for the red reflex—a reflex dilatation of the blood vessels on the handle of the malleus caused by the otoscope speculum touching the bony ear canal. Also, a crying child will often have flushed, erythematous tympanic membranes (TM). This is often misdiagnosed as early acute otitis media, and the true cause of otalgia is missed. Always consider if the otalgia is referred pain.

History	Examination (using an otoscope)	Diagnosis	Page no.
Severe pain Child/preceding URI Very painful Aural fullness and decreased hearing	Erythema—a bulging tympanic membrane Temperature	Acute otitis media Bullous myringitis	258
Severe pain Preceding itch Long-standing Surfer/swimmer	Narrow EAC Osteoma Mucopus Painful auricle	Otitis externa Look for foreign body	242
Severe pain Elderly	EAC floor with granulation tissue Cranial nerve palsies	Necrotizing otitis externa	244
Intermittent severe pain At night time History of recurrent otitis media Aural fullness and hearing loss Chronic symptoms	Middle ear effusion	Glue ear Cholesteotoma	261

Additional history annotations:
- Not diabetic and normal immune system → (Otitis externa)
- Diabetic / HIV / Immunocompromised → (Necrotizing otitis externa)

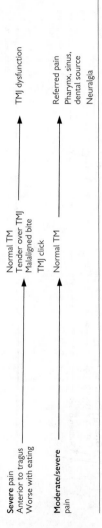

Severe pain
Anterior to tragus
Worse with eating

→ Normal TM
Tender over TMJ
Malaligned bite
TMJ click

→ TMJ dysfunction

Moderate/severe
pain

→ Normal TM

→ Referred pain
Pharynx, sinus,
dental source
Neuralgia

Hearing loss

A diagnosis of hearing loss in children and adults depends on combining the information from the patient's history, the examination, and any special investigations. An audiogram, or a tympanogram with tuning-fork tests will help to distinguish conductive from sensorineural hearing loss and will determine if the problem is bilateral or affects only one ear.

Sudden hearing loss is an emergency.

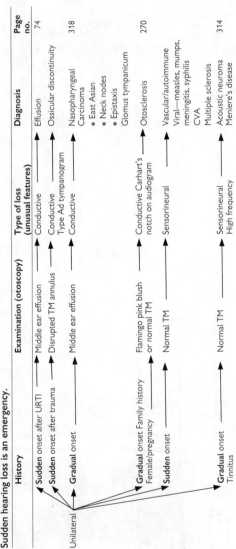

	History	Examination (otoscopy)	Type of loss (unusual features)	Diagnosis	Page no.
	Sudden onset after URTI	Middle ear effusion	Conductive	Effusion	74
	Sudden onset after trauma	Disrupted TM annulus	Conductive Type Ad tympanogram	Ossicular discontinuity	
Unilateral	**Gradual** onset	Middle ear effusion	Conductive	Nasopharyngeal Carcinoma • East Asian • Neck nodes • Epistaxis Glomus tympanicum	318
	Gradual onset Family history Female/pregnancy	Flamingo pink blush or normal TM	Conductive Carhart's notch on audiogram	Otosclerosis	270
	Sudden onset	Normal TM	Sensorineural	Vascular/autoimmune Viral—measles, mumps, meningitis, syphilis CVA Multiple sclerosis	
	Gradual onset Tinnitus	Normal TM	Sensorineural High frequency	Acoustic neuroma Meniere's disease	314

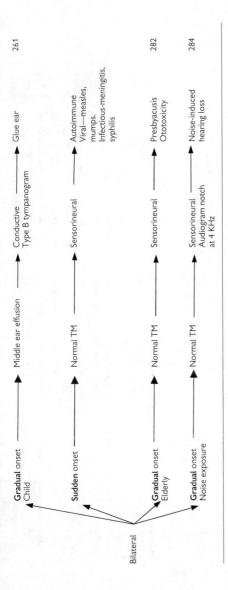

Bilateral

Gradual onset
Child → Middle ear effusion → Conductive
Type B tympanogram → Glue ear   261

Sudden onset → Normal TM → Sensorineural → Autoimmune
Viral—measles,
mumps.
Infectious-meningitis,
syphilis

Gradual onset
Elderly → Normal TM → Sensorineural → Presbyacusis
Ototoxicity   282

Gradual onset
Noise exposure → Normal TM → Sensorineural
Audiogram notch
at 4 KHz → Noise-induced
hearing loss   284

Tinnitus

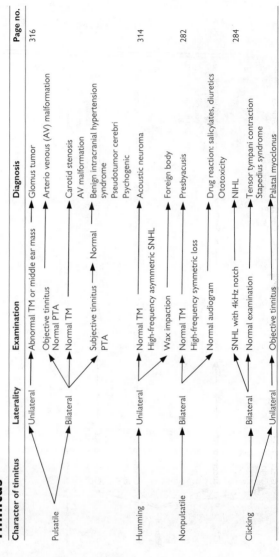

Character of tinnitus	Laterality	Examination	Diagnosis	Page no.
Pulsatile	Unilateral	Abnormal TM or middle ear mass	Glomus tumor	316
			Arterio venous (AV) malformation	
	Bilateral	Objective tinnitus Normal PTA	Carotid stenosis AV malformation	
		Normal TM		
		Subjective tinnitus PTA → Normal	Benign intracranial hypertension syndrome Pseudotumor cerebri Psychogenic	
Humming	Unilateral	Normal TM High-frequency asymmetric SNHL	Acoustic neuroma	314
		Wax impaction	Foreign body	
Nonpulsatile	Bilateral	Normal TM High-frequency symmetric loss	Presbyacusis	282
		Normal audiogram	Drug reaction: salicylates, diuretics Ototoxicity	
		SNHL with 4kHz notch	NIHL	284
Clicking	Bilateral	Normal examination	Tensor tympani contraction Stapedius syndrome	
	Unilateral	Objective tinnitus	Palatal myoclonus	

Facial pain

Patients with this problem may present to a variety of specialties for an opinion, e.g., ENT, neurology, or maxillofacial surgery.

History	Examination	Diagnosis	Page no.
Severe acute pain Pain periorbital/cheeks Provoked by URTI Nasal obstruction Temperature	Pus/polyps in middle meatus →	Acute sinusitis Dacrocystitis	123
Chronic fullness Worse bending over Nasal obstruction	Middle meatus occluded/narrowed → CT scan findings of sinus mucosal thickening	Chronic sinusitis	125
Severe pain Localized to specific site No nasal obstruction No nasal symptoms	Normal nasal examination → Normal nasal endoscopy	Migraines Tension headaches Postherpetic neuralgia Trigeminal neuralgia Temporal arteritis Atypical facial pain Glaucoma Sialolithiasis or sialoadenitis	
Intermittent pain Worse on eating Radiates to ear	Normal nasal examination → Normal nasal endoscopy Tenderness over TMJ	TMJ dysfunction Bruxism	

Investigations in ENT

Hearing physiology

Hearing is the product of a special sensory pathway that involves the detection of sound energy through air vibration that gets transformed into neuroelectrical signals for interpretation by the brain. The physiology and anatomy of hearing is reviewed in detail in Chapters 12 to 14. The sound energy is propagated through the air and collected in the external ear. The external ear is designed to collected and funnel sound towards the eardrum or tympanic membrane. The tympanic membrane then collects the air vibrations and transforms them into mechanical vibration towards the inner ear via the middle ear bones, or ossicles. The ossicular chain is composed of three bones, the malleus, incus, and stapes. The stapes articulates with the inner ear cochlea via the stapes footplate and distributes the vibration into the fluid-filled spaces of the cochlea. Inner hair cells of the cochlea depolarize in response to the fluid wave and send the sound signal into the brainstem via the auditory nerve, a component of cranial nerve 8. This signal goes to the dorsal cochlear nucleus, which then distributes the neural signal to the temporal lobe via the thalamus.

At each step of the process of translating and transforming the air-conducted vibratory sound energy into neural signal, there are special adaptations of the hearing apparatus. The pinna and the external auditory canal have a natural resonance of approximately 2000 Hz and are responsible for a gain of approximately 20 dB. The size of the tympanic membrane in comparison to the stapes footplate is approximately 15 to 1, resulting in a 15-fold amplification. The lever action of the middle ear ossicles further amplifies the vibration 1.3-fold. The net amplification is 20-fold, which results in a gain of approximately 20 to 35 dB.

The audiogram is composed of several parts designed to test the various components of hearing. Air tone audiometry is used to test the entire pathway from the external ear to the brain, while bone conduction tests the pathway from the inner ear function onward. Otoacoustic emissions testing is used to look specifically at cochlear function, and auditory brainstem testing evaluates the auditory nerve pathway towards the brain. Tympanometry tests the tympanic membrane resistance. By using these tests and understanding the physiology of the auditory system, otolaryngologists can diagnose the location of ear problems.

Definitions

Bell (B) Unit of sound intensity and pressure.

Decibel (dB) 10 Bell. A decibel is a *relative* measure. Zero dB is set as the lowest intensity of sound an average normal ear can detect. A decibel is a *nonlinear* measurement. The difference between 1 and 2 dB is 10-fold.

Pure tone audiometry (PTA)

This is the most common method used for assessing hearing. Ideally, the examination takes place in a soundproof booth. The ears should be clear of any obstructing cerumen.

The examiner and the patient are in contact via a microphone and a headset. The patient wears headphones and is given a handheld button to press when he or she hears a sound during the test. The better hearing ear is tested first.

The test begins with air-conducted sounds. Initially, sound is played through the headphones at a level above the hearing threshold. The sound is decreased in 10 dB increments until it is no longer heard. The sound intensity is then increased in 5 dB increments until a 50% response rate is obtained.

- The frequency order of testing is 1 kHz, 2 kHz, 4 kHz, 8 kHz, 500 Hz, 250 Hz, and then repeated at 1 kHz.
- The re-test at 1 kHz should be within 10 dB of the initial result.
- The test–retest error is approximately 5 dB.

The test is then repeated using bone conduction. The bone conductor is tightly applied to the mastoid area where the skin is tethered to the bone more securely and better contact is obtained. Sound is transmitted to the cochlea as direct vibration of the temporal bone. Because the vibrations are easily transmitted to the opposite temporal bone, *masking* is frequently required. The bone conduction studies are compared with the air conduction studies to obtain the air bone gap. Whereas air conduction studies test the entire auditory tract, the bone conduction studies bypass the external and middle ear components and directly test the cochlear function and downstream components.

Interpretation of pure tone audiometry

- Normal hearing is detection of pure tones at less than 20 dB.
- Mild hearing loss: 21–40 dB
- Moderate hearing loss: 41–60 dB
- Severe hearing loss: 61–80 dB
- Profound hearing loss: no detection of pure tones below 81 dB

Masking

Like tuning-fork testing, there is a potential source of error in the pure tone audiogram. This is because sound can be perceived in the non-test ear if it is conducted through bone or through the air. The main differences are the following:

- 10 dB for bone conduction
- 40 dB for air conduction

When thresholds show a difference of >10 dB or >40 dB, then masking should be used. This is the amount of sound intensity detectable to the opposite ear when a sound is presented to one ear.

Masking is the application of white noise to the non-test ear to prevent it from picking up sounds presented to the test ear. Masking is required when

- Air conduction audiometry shows a >40 dB difference in the two ears.
- The difference in air conduction threshold between the test ear and the bone conduction in the non-test ear is >40 dB.
- An unmasked air bone gap in the test ear is >10 dB (a sensorineural loss may be hidden).

Speech audiometry

Speech reception is an important component of the audiogram and evaluates the ability to interpret sound energy and process it into recognizable patterns. In speech audiometry, spoken words, generally balanced monosyllabic words (phonemes) or two-syllable words (spondees), are used.

Definitions

Pure tone average (PTA) The average thresholds for the most important speech frequencies, 500, 1000, and 2000 HZ.

Speech reception threshold (SRT) The lowest decibel of hearing that a patient can repeat a spondee 50% of the time. The SRT should be within 10 dB of the PTA.

Speech Discrimination Score (SDS) The percentage (%) of phonemes that the patient can repeat correctly at 20 to 40 dB above the SRT.

Rollover A phenomenon that reflects the ability of a retrocochlear process to cause greater problems with discrimination. Patients have a poor SRT and SDS disproportionate to their PTA.

Tympanometry

Tympanometry is a way of measuring the pressure in the middle ear. It was developed and popularized by Jerger[1] as a way of establishing the cause of conductive deafness. He classified the different patterns described later (see Fig. 4.1).

Method

A probe is placed in the external auditory meatus to give a tight seal to the external ear canal (EAC). This probe can vary the pressure in the EAC while firing a 225 Hz sound signal at the tympanic membrane (TM), or eardrum. The probe then measures the amount of sound reflected from the TM and calculates how much of the sound energy is admitted. Most sound is admitted when the pressure in the EAC matches that of the middle ear space. Thus, the instrument measures the compliance of the TM. By calculating the amount of air needed to change the EAC pressure, the machine also calculates an approximate EAC volume.

Normal ear

Type A Normal tympanogram. The peak is at atmospheric pressure and reflects maximal compliance.

Ossicular chain problems

Type As (A shallow) The normal tympanogram can be flattened as a fixed ossicular chain reduces compliance. This can be the result of otosclerosis or middle ear effusion.

Type Ad (A deep) The disarticulated ossicular chain causes the compliance to increase. This can also occur with a thinned-out or monomeric tympanic membrane.

Middle ear effusion or glue ear

Type B When there is fluid in the middle ear, the ear drum's compliance alters, giving a flat trace.

Perforation

Type B If there is a perforation in the tympanic membrane, the compliance will remain unchanged. But EAC volume will be increased as the tympanometer measures the pressure of the EAC and middle ear space.

Eustachian tube dysfunction

Type C The peak of the tympanogram is shifted to the left side. This type is often associated with eustachian tube dysfunction.

1 Jerger J. (1970). Clinical experience with impedance audiometry. *Arch Otolaryngol* **92**:311–24.

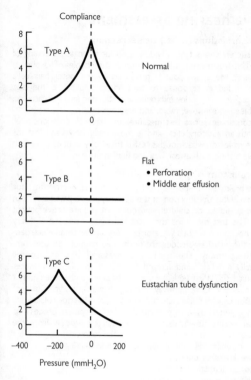

Fig. 4.1 Types of tympanogram.

Objective hearing assessment

Otoacoustic emissions (OAE) test screening

The otoacoustic emissions test is widely used for neonatal screening of hearing loss. This test measures the function of the cochlea. This phenomenon measures the active sounds produced by the outer hair cells which are recorded in response to tone clicks applied to the ear. The sound is picked up by a tiny microphone embedded into the earpiece. The test is objective, sensitive, rapid, and easy to perform. The transient-evoked otoacoustic emissions test measures the hair cell emissions after stimulation with an auditory click, and is most commonly used test for screening. The major drawback of this test is that many entities can result in false positive testing, such as ear wax and fluid in the ear.

Auditory brainstem response

The auditory brainstem response (ABR) is another objective test for hearing that evaluates the function of the auditory nerve pathway. It can be performed on adults or children and does not require active patient cooperation. The test measures the electrical signal from the auditory nerve to the brain with various waveforms. Very similar to an electroencephalogram, the signal electrodes are positioned to measure the components of the pathway. The signals are measured after an acoustic stimulus, usually a "click," and filtered to record specific ABR waves. The mneumonic E.COLI is frequently used to help remember the components of the auditory nerve pathway: the **E**ighth cranial nerve, **C**ochlear nucleus, superior **O**livary nuclei, lateral **L**emniscus, and **I**nferior colliculus.

The ABR is generally used to evaluate for a retrocochlear process, or pathology that occurs downstream of the auditory process from the cochlea. Various common uses of ABR include the following:
• Asymmetric or unilateral auditory process such as hearing loss, vestibular weakness, or tinnitus
• Screening for an acoustic neuroma
• Children who failed auditory screening
• Suspected malingerers
• Coma
• Intraoperative monitoring

Pediatric hearing assessment

Congenital hearing loss affects approximately 1 in every 1000 newborns. Screening based on risk factors alone may miss up to 42% of hearing-impaired infants. Universal screening is endorsed by the American Academy of Pediatrics, the National Institutes of Health, and the Centers for Disease Control and Prevention.

Risk factors for hearing loss include the presence of craniofacial abnormalities, a positive family history of childhood hearing loss, neonatal intensive care unit admission for longer than 2 days, fetal infections such as cytomegalovirus (CMV), rubella, or herpes, and presence of other syndromes associated with hearing loss such as Usher's or Wallenburg's syndrome. All neonates with these risk factors should be tested.

Assessment of the hearing of infants and children can be difficult because most hearing tests involve the active cooperation of the participant. To avoid this problem, a number of tests have been specifically designed for children and different tests are used at different ages. Objective testing such as otoacoustic emissions and auditory brainstem testing are very useful in the early stages. OAE testing is the most common screening program for neonates.

Distraction testing

Two testers are required for this examination. The child sits on the parent or caregiver's lap, and one of the examiners sits in front of the child to occupy the child's attention. The other tester stands behind the child and uses sounds of particular frequency and volume to stimulate the child to turn the head. Turning is considered a positive response.

Visual reinforcement audiometry

This test is similar to distraction testing, but it uses speakers or headphones to deliver the unilateral sound. If the child turns around correctly, then a light or a toy turns on to reward their turning.

Conditioned response audiometry

The child is conditioned to perform a task in response to a sound—for example, putting a toy man into a toy boat.

McCormick toy testing

This test uses 12 paired toys or objects with similar-sounding names, for example, a cup and a duck. The child points to or picks up the correct toy. The intensity of the sound of the command can be changed. The child's hearing threshold is determined by an 80% response.

Pure tone audiogram

This can sometimes be performed on children as young as 3 years of age. Use of PTA with bone conduction can be uncomfortable for younger children.

Tympanometry

This test measures pressure in the middle ear and is useful and accurate in detecting middle-ear effusions in children.

Electronystagmography (ENG)

Electronystagmography (ENG) is a balance test that measures the chorioretinal electrical potential difference. Electrodes placed near the eyes can pick up electrical changes caused by eye movements. ENG allows testing of the vestibulo-ocular reflex (VOR). The VOR enables clear vision during head movements by producing compensatory eye movements.

The ENG test is usually done in a dimly lit room with a light bar to provide visual calibration. The patient sits on an examination couch.

Uses of ENG

ENG enables an assessment of the following:
- Disorders in semicircular canal (SCC) and otolith organs
- Integrity of brainstem–cerebellar pathways
- Integrity of central vestibulo-ocular pathways

Subtests

If patients need more detailed investigations, they may be sent for more tests, which may include:
- Oculomotor control test
  - Saccades
  - Tracking/smooth pursuit
  - Optokinetic test
  - Gaze test
- Positional testing
  - Headshake
  - Dix–Hallpike test
- Caloric tests
  - Warm and cold irrigations
  - Ice calorics
  - Fixation tests

Calorics

This balance test involves irrigating warm or cold water into the ear. This stimulates the inner-ear balance mechanisms and will make the patient dizzy. The degree of stimulation can be measured by observing the nystagmus produced. This test is performed on both ears, and any difference gives an indication of pathology in the balance system. It is used to confirm an inner-ear cause of a balance problem.

Procedure

- Irrigation with warm water at 44°C and cool at 30°C the EAC for 30 seconds with 200 ml of fluid
- Alternatively warm air at 50°C and cool at 24°C for 60 seconds at 9 L/min flow rate
- Temperature difference stimulates convection currents in the lateral SCC. Nystagmus is induced according to the mneumonic COWS (Cold Opposite, Warm the Same). Cold induces an opposite-sided nystagmus, while warmth induces nystagmus toward the same side. Remember, nystagmus is named by the fast component.
- Responses are compared according to formula below.

Unilateral weakness (>25% significance)

$$\frac{(RC + RW) - (LC + LW) \times 100}{RC + LC + RW + LW} = \text{unilateral weakness}$$

Directional preponderance (>25%–30% significance)

$$\frac{(RC + RW) - (LC + RW) \times 100}{RC + LC + RW + LW} = \text{directional preponderance}$$

where RC = Right Cold
       RW = Right Warm
       LC = Left Cold
       LW = Left Warm

CT scan

Computed tomography (CT) provides excellent information for defining differences between bone and soft tissue. Non-contrast CT scans allow very precise imaging of bony structures within the head and neck as well as air spaces. Non-contrast CT is commonly used to look for problems affecting the temporal bone and the inner ear, the paranasal sinuses, facial bones, and the upper airway. The addition of intravenous contrast enables the evaluation of soft-tissue structures in the neck, which is important for detecting head and neck tumors and cancers as well as infection. CT angiograms show precise delineation of vascular structures and can be used for the evaluation of uncontrollable bleeding, vascular tumors and anomalies, aortic dissections, and thrombosis.

Procedure

The patient lies supine on the scanner bed. The scan uses X-rays applied in a circumferential manner to acquire cross-sectional information, which is processed and formatted to produce images. These can be manipulated to form images in multiple planes or to produce three-dimensional reconstructions.

Specific imaging protocols that detail the slice thickness, plane and angle of imaging (gantry), administration of contrast, and area scanned need to be specified. Generally, the specific details are ordered by the radiologist according to the diagnosis being evaluated. Therefore, a protocol for the evaluation of sinus disease is different from that needed for the evaluation of temporal bone fractures.

Common uses

• Paranasal sinus scan is used to evaluate chronic and acute sinusitis and for detailing the bony anatomy for endoscopic sinus surgery.
• Evaluation of head and neck masses.
• Evaluation of the deep extension of mucosal disease as well as lymphadenopathy.
• Assessment of middle ear and mastoid infections.
• Assessment of temporal bone and skull base for infections and tumors.
• Evaluation of traumatic head, neck, and facial injuries and temporal bone fracture.

MRI scan

Magnetic resonance imaging (MRI) provides excellent soft-tissue definition without the risk of radiation. In Otolaryngology it is used for looking at soft-tissue structures such as the nerves of the inner ear and for differentiating neoplastic disease from normal structures. In magnetic angiography (MRA) special computer filters are used to extract images of blood flow, and thus MRA can be used for the evaluation of vascular structures. Evaluation of bony anatomy as well as air-bone interface is more difficult with MRI than with CT scanning.

Procedure

The patient is placed lying down, inside a circular magnet. The magnetic field aligns all the hydrogen atoms, mainly body water. An electromagnetic pulse is directed toward the patient, which knocks the hydrogen atoms out of alignment. Once the pulse wave has subsided, the hydrogen atoms spring back into alignment. This process causes energy to be released, which is detected by the scanner.

The timing of recording and the information collected can be analyzed separately to give different information. Software algorithms can be used to produce three-dimensional (3D) image information. Contrast with gadolinium can enhance the information. Gadolinium is a paramagnetic metal ion used as a contrast agent to provide additional information about the vascularity of a structure.

Contraindications to MRI include ferromagnetic implants such as intracranial aneurysm clips, cardiac pacemakers, some cochlear implants, and middle-ear prosthetics.

Common protocols

- T1-weighted scans (fat bright)
- T2-weighted scans (water bright)
- STIR sequence (short tau inversion recovery) produces fat-suppressed images.
- MRA information from scan sequence

Uses

- Identifying an acoustic neuroma—MRI is the gold standard
- Checking the spread of a tumor
- Assessing the involvement of vascular structures in head and neck malignancy
- Assessing the intracranial spread for sinonasal and skull base tumors

PET scan

In positron emission tomography (PET) a radioactive marker is used that measures the amount of glucose consumed in a specific structure. Although its utility is expanding, PET scanning is most commonly used for the evaluation of neoplastic disease. 18-F-fluorodeoxyglucose (FDG) is concentrated in structures with a high glycolytic rate, such as tumors and infections. PET scans are very sensitive for picking up inflammation and are not specific for tumors.

Common uses

- Evaluation of an unknown primary tumor in patients with metastatic neck cancer
- Assessment of residual or recurrent disease following therapy or in a postsurgical bed
- Search for synchronous or metachronous primary lesions
- Search for metastatic disease, especially distant metastases

Skin prick testing

This test enables you to detect if a patient is allergic to various substances. It has a rapid result, allowing you to see the allergic response. Skin prick testing is used in patients with allergic rhinitis, to guide therapy and to give advice on which allergens to avoid. The test relies on histamine release by sensitized mast cells. Antihistamines, steroids, and certain other medications (calcium channel blockers and tricyclic antidepressants) may decrease the sensitivity of the test.

Intradermal testing is similar in technique and use to skin prick testing, except the injection is placed deeper and at higher concentrations. This results in greater sensitivity at higher risk for anaphylaxis.

Procedure

- Because of the risk for anaphylaxis during skin prick testing, it is important to ensure that resuscitation facilities are nearby.
- The procedure for testing should be explained to the patient. The test solutions are then placed on the patient's forearm. These include a positive control substance (histamine) and a negative control substance (carrier solution). A small amount of solution is inoculated by using a lancet pricked into the patient's skin.
- A positive response is measured after 15–30 minutes, as a wheal >4 mm. (It should be at least 2 mm greater than the negative control.)

The mouth, tonsils, and adenoids

Anatomy

The oral cavity extends from the lips to the anterior pillar of the tonsil (see Fig. 5.1). The superior extent is marked at the hard palate and soft palate junction while the inferior boundary is marked by the circumvallate papilla of the tongue. Subsites include the lips, the inferior and superior alveolar ridges, anterior tongue, floor of mouth, retromolar trigone, hard palate, and buccal mucosa.

The oropharynx extends from the anterior tonsillar pillar to the posterior pharyngeal wall. The superior junction is at the interface of the hard and soft palate while the inferior junction is marked at the circumvallate papilla. The oropharynx contains the tonsils, soft palate, lateral pharyngeal walls, and the base of the tongue.

The nasopharynx is located above the hard palate and contains the adenoids. The torus tubarius encloses the eustachian tubes orifices laterally. The superior lateral extent is marked by the fossa of Rosenmuller and the base of the sphenoid. The nasopharynx communicates with the nasal cavity anteriorly. The soft palate forms the inferior boundary.

The tongue

The anterior two-thirds and posterior third of the tongue have different embryological origins and different nerve supplies. The junction is at the sulcus terminalis, which is marked by the circumvallate papillae.

Motor supply to the tongue is via the hypoglossal nerve (CN12).

Sensation to the anterior two-thirds of the tongue is via the lingual nerve (CN5). The posterior third is supplied by the glossopharyngeal nerve (CN9).

Taste fibers travel with the facial nerve (CN7) towards the middle ear. The chorda typani carries the special sensory of taste fibers and exits the middle ear to merge with the mandibular division of the trigeminal nerve. At the tongue, the fibers are incorporated within the lingual nerve.

Muscles of the tongue The motion of the tongue is very complex and is composed of sets of intrinsic and extrinsic muscles. The intrinsic muscles do not have bony attachments and are aligned in different vectors to alter the shape of the tongue. The extrinsic muscles move the tongue and have attachments to the mandible, the styloid process, and the hyoid bone. The extrinsic muscles are the genioglossus, hyoglossus, and styloglossus.

The palate

The palate consists of a bony hard palate composed primarily of maxillary bone and a muscular soft palate. The palate serves to divide and separate the mouth from the nose. The soft palate has a role in phonation, assists in the patency of the eustachian tube, and forms a seal during deglutination. Patients with velopharyngeal insufficiency complain of nasal regurgitation of food during eating. The muscles of the soft palate include the tensor veli palatine, the levator veli palatine, palatoglossus, and the palatopharyngeus. There is also a small muscle in the uvula called the musculus uvula. All the muscles of the palate are innervated by the vagus nerve, with the notable exception of the tensor veli palatini, which is innervated by the mandibular branch of the trigeminal nerve CN5.

Waldeyer's ring

The mouth is a continuation of the gastrointestinal tract and is the primary entry point for many potential pathogens. *Waldeyer's ring* refers to the ring of lymphoid tissue that circumferentially lines the oropharynx and nasopharynx. The ring is composed of the paired palatine tonsils, the pharyngeal tonsils or adenoids, and the lingual tonsils. Waldeyer's ring generally begins to proliferate from 1 to 3 years of age and peaks at around age 5. During this period, it is common to get obstructive symptoms related to adenotonsillar hypertrophy. After puberty, the lymphoid tissues begin to regress.

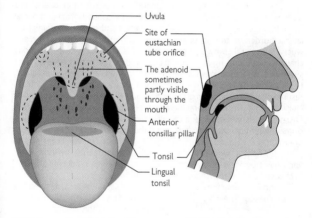

Fig. 5.1 Anteroposterior view of oral cavity and lateral view of oropharynx and nasopharynx.

Oral ulcers—benign

Traumatic ulcers

Acute traumatic ulcers heal quickly and rarely require medical attention. Chronic traumatic ulcers are seen quite often. These can arise from ill-fitting dentures or sharp or rotten teeth, and usually occur on the lateral aspect of the tongue, or on the inside of the cheek. Treatment consists of dental review or refitting of the denture.

Aphthous ulcers

These common mouth ulcers, otherwise known as canker sores, start to appear usually during childhood or adolescence as round or oval ulcerations with well-circumscribed margins, erythematous borders, and gray or yellow centers. They are small and painful and most often affect the lateral border or the tip of the tongue, although they may occur anywhere in the oral cavity. The exact etiology is unclear, although hormonal changes, poor oral hygiene, trauma, poor diet, and stress have all been suggested as factors. Predisposing factors include hematologic deficiency (such as iron, folic acid, or vitamin B) in up to 20% of patients; gastrointestinal disorders causing malabsorption; and chronic exposure to sodium lauryl sulfate, a common ingredient in oral health-care products. Drugs such as nonsteroidal anti-inflammatory drugs (NSAIDS) and alendronate have also been implicated. Aphthous ulcers also occur in Crohn's disease; celiac disease; Neumann bipolar aphthosis (genital ulcers may be present); Behcet syndrome; HIV infection; neutropenia; periodic fever, aphthous stomatitis, pharyngitis, and cervical adenitis syndrome (PFAPA) in children; and Sweet syndrome.

Aphthous ulcers affect 5%–66% of the population, with a slight female predominance. They typically heal in 7–10 days. Occasionally they are severe and recurrent and last longer. Treatment in this case should consist of simple analgesia, local anesthetic gels, or topical steroid. Topical corticosteroids can help with the symptoms but do not reduce the rate of recurrence. Commonly used preparations include trimaicinolone acetonide in carboxymethyl cellulose paste (Adcortyl in orabase, Kenlaog) applied four times a day. Rarely, a single giant aphthous ulcer may develop. Occasionally, biopsy may be necessary to distinguish between a long-standing ulcer and malignancy. Care should be taken to biopsy the border of the ulcer to obtain a portion of intact epithelium for histologic evaluation.

Infective ulcers

Herpes labialis can be caused by herpes simplex virus (HSV) I and HSV II. Primary infection is usually asymptomatic. For those who are symptomatic, gingivostomatitis and pharyngitis are common. Lesions around the mouth can also occur. Typical signs of the initial infection are fever, malaise, mylagia, and cervical adenopathy lasting 3–14 days. After a latency period, reactivation can occur in 20%–40% of people and is characterized by vesicles and ulcerations around the mouth, known as cold sores or fever blisters. Ulcerations can occur inside the mouth, on the lips, or on the face.

When herpes labialis occurs inside the mouth, it can be confused with aphthous ulcers. Herpes labialis tends to recur in the same place, in contrast to aphthous ulcers, which occur in different places. There is usually a prodrome preceding reactivated HSV episodes, with tingling, pain, and erythema occurring at the site. Precipitating factors include ultraviolet (UV) light, fever, stress, premenstruation, and procedures affecting the site such as dental or oral surgery, injections, or laser procedures. Before such surgical procedures, premedication with acyclovir may be recommended, especially in those with a history of cold sores.

Herpes labialis is transmitted through direct contact with skin. The highest chance of transmission of the virus is when there is an active lesion present.

Diagnosis is made on the basis of clinical presentation. Oral treatment consists of acyclovir or valacyclovir. Valacyclovir 2 g bid for 1 day has been demonstrated to shorten healing time and pain during recurrent episodes. Acyclovir 200–400 mg five times a day for 5 days and Famvir 500 mg tid for 5 days can also be given. If a person develops frequent reactivations, chronic suppression treatment may be considered.

Another infectious cause of mouth lesions is syphilis, caused by *Treponema pallidum.* Primary syphilis usually presents as a painless ulceration in the genitalia ("chancre") and rarely may present in the mouth. Secondary syphilis, with its more protean manisfestations (syphilis is often referred to as the "great imitator") can occur as small papules on the corner of the mouth, known as "split papules." The treatment of choice is penicillin.

Dietary and blood disorders

Ulcerative stomatitis is often the product of underlying systemic disorders. Deficiencies in iron, folate, and vitamin B_{12} can cause oral ulceration, since these agents are required for normal mucosal development. Mouth ulcers also occur as a result of leukemia, polycythemia, and agranulocytosis.

Signs of scurvy and pellagra include a sore mouth and ulceration. These ulcerations are generally larger and more widespread. Behcet syndrome is a poorly understood systemic disorder involving recurrent oral ulcers and either eye, skin, or genital ulcerations.

Systemic disorders

The mouth is a continuation of the gastrointestinal tract and can have ulcerations as part of inflammatory bowel disease. Conditions associated with drug allergies such as Stevens Johnson syndrome have oral ulcerations.

Torus palatinus

This is a benign osteoma on the hard palate. Its surface may become ulcerated, usually as a result of trauma. In this case the lesion may look and feel malignant. These lesions need only be removed if they repeatedly become infected or interfere with the fitting of a dental plate.

Oral ulcers—malignant

Squamous cell carcinoma (SCC)

This is the most common malignant lesion found in the mouth. The appearance can vary considerably and range from erythematous patches to exophytic ulcerations. The primary risk factors are tobacco (smoking and chewing) and alcohol use. Other risk factors include chewing betel nuts and poor oral hygiene. Viral risk factors include the presence of HSV and human papilloma virus. There is an estimated annual incidence of 30,000 new oral cancers with approximately 4800 deaths per year in the United States.

Symptoms and signs

Squamous cell carcinomas are lesions of the mucosal epithelium. The appearance can vary but they often look irregular and keratotic with areas of ulceration. These ulcers progress and may become painful, often with referred pain to the ear. Pain often denotes invasion or infiltration into adjacent sensory nerves or infection. Malignant ulcers of the tongue may be superficial or deeply infiltrating. They usually feel firm and irregular to palpation. Other symptoms include difficulty swallowing and weight loss or a neck mass.

Investigations

More information can usually be gathered from palpation than from inspection. It is vital to adequately examine the neck for lymph node metastasis, paying particular attention to the submandibular and submental triangles as well as those nodes deep to the sternomastoid running along the internal jugular vein. SCC of the oral cavity will most commonly metastasize to the nodes in levels 1, 2, and 3 (see p. 102). An MRI or CT scan is most often used to assess the neck. A finding of enlarged lymph nodes greater than 1–1.5 cm in the presence of known SCC is usually sufficient to warrant neck dissection. In skilled hands, ultrasound-guided FNA is a highly sensitive and specific tool in assessing the neck.

Management

Any ulcer that fails to heal within 2 weeks should be biopsied to exclude malignancy. Many patients who develop oral-cavity SCC have widespread mucosal-field change as a result of their smoking and drinking. They are at a high risk of developing another upper aerodigestive tract cancer at the same time or at some time in the future. All patients presenting with SCC should have a panendoscopy under general anesthetic to exclude any additional primary tumor. The panendoscopy will also allow proper assessment of the primary tumor.

Treatment

Treatment and management of oral SCC are dependent on tumor size, lymph node spread, and presence of distant metastasis. The American Joint Commission on Cancer (AJCC) uses a T, N, M staging method for head and neck cancer (Table 5.1). Options include external beam and interstitial radiotherapy as well as surgical en-bloc resection. The surgically created defect will require reconstruction to produce an acceptable functional and cosmetic result for the patient.

Table 5.1 Oral cavity primary tumor staging

T0	No evidence of primary tumor
T1	Tumor <2 cm
T2	Tumor 2–4 cm
T3	Tumor >4 cm
T4	Tumor invades surrounding structures such as cortical bone, extrinsic muscles of the tongue, skin, and maxillary sinus

From 1997 TNM staging system, American Joint Committee on Cancer (AJCC)

White patches in the mouth

There are many possible causes of white patches in the mouth. These causes are described below.

Candida

Candida tends to occur in debilitated and immunocompromised patients. White specs coalesce to form patches, or a white membrane, which when lifted reveals a red, raw mucosal surface. It sometimes occurs on the soft palate and can complicate the use of steroid inhalers in asthma patients. Candida is usually diagnosed by seeing it, but if any doubt remains, scrapings of the lesion should be taken and sent for microbiological examination.

Leukoplakia

Although any white patch in the mouth can be called leukoplakia, the term usually refers to hyperkeratosis of the oral mucosa. This happens to patients who share the same risk factors as those who develop SCC: smoking, alcohol, and prolonged irritation from sharp teeth or poorly fitting dentures. This lesion is premalignant and 3% of patients will undergo malignant change within 5 years of diagnosis. A biopsy and regular reviews are essential.

A particular form of leukoplakia known as oral hairy leukoplakia occurs in immunocompromised and immunocompetent HIV patients. It may also occur in HIV-negative patients who have hematologic malignancies. The condition is thought to be caused by the Epstein–Barr virus and appears as painless white plaques on the lateral aspect of the tongue. They may be smooth or hairy or feathery with prominent projections. They frequently appear and disappear spontaneously.

Oral lichen planus

This T-cell-mediated autoimmune condition occurs on the buccal mucosa, gingiva, and tongue. Onset is typically during adulthood, with a female predilection and association with other autoimmune diseases such as alopecia areata, dermatomyositis, lichen sclerosus et atrophicus, or primary biliary cirrhosis. Lesions have a white, reticulated, lace-like appearance. Ulcerations or erosions may be present. Two-thirds of cases may be extremely painful, especially if lesions are ulcerative. Thalidomide has been reported to be a successful treatment.

Mucus retention cysts

These cysts usually form a smooth, pale, round protuberance and can occur anywhere in the oral cavity, base of the tongue, or tonsils. These swellings arise from a blockage in one of the many mucus glands found throughout the mucosa of the upper aerodigestive tract. Reassurance is usually all that is required. If there is any diagnostic uncertainty, or if they become large enough to cause symptoms, excision or marsupialization may be required.

Miscellaneous mouth conditions

Geographic tongue

Also known as benign migratory glossitis, this is a common, benign condition that occurs in 3% of the population. Atrophy of the filiform papillae results in red patches with a white border. Although lesions are usually asymptomatic, some patients have noted increased sensitivity to hot and spicy food. The sites of predilection vary and seem to move around the tongue. The cause is unknown, but it often runs in families and there is an increased prevalence among people with psoriasis. Reassurance is the only treatment required.

Angioedema

This allergic reaction causes generalized swelling of the tongue. Seafood, peanuts, and drugs such as angiotensin-converting enzyme (ACE) inhibitors can all have this effect. The swelling may progress rapidly and obstruct the airway. Medical treatment consists of intravenous steroids, diphenhydramine, and racemic epinephrine. The airway may need to be secured by either endotracheal intubation or tracheotomy.

Median rhomboid glossitis

This appears as a raised, smooth plaque in the center of the dorsum of the tongue. It has been linked with reflux and candida infection. In most cases, simple reassurance is all that is required. Antifungal treatment can be helpful to reduce redness and inflammation associated with candida infection. Some lesions disappear after antifungal therapy.

Tongue tie

Ankyloglossia is a birth defect in which tongue movement is restricted due to the abnormal attachment of the base of the tongue toward the tip of the tongue. This condition is often hereditary. Tongue tie can cause feeding problems in infants. In some children, it can cause speech problems. Surgical division can be easily performed in the office with few adverse effects.

Macroglossia

Enlargement of the tongue can be seen in acromegaly, Down syndrome, multiple endocrine adenoma syndrome, hypothyroidism, and amyloidosis.

Burning tongue syndrome

Patients with this condition complain of a burning sensation of the tongue, lips, gums, palate, throat, or throughout the mouth. It tends to occur in middle-aged to older adults, with a higher frequency among women. Its cause is unknown and treatment is tailored to the individual on the basis of specific underlying etiology, such as xerostomia (dryness), infectious causes such as thrush, or psychological factors.

Hairy oral leukoplakia

This condition appears as white patches on the lateral border of the tongue in patients with AIDS.

Black hairy tongue

This aptly named condition occurs from overgrowth of the filiform papillae of the tongue and generally occurs in smokers. Treatment consists of brushing the tongue with a soft toothbrush.

Ranula

This is a retention cyst that forms in the floor of the mouth under the tongue. It develops from the submandibular or sublingual glands. It is treated by marsupialization and removal of the adjacent sublingual gland.

Cystic hygroma

This is a benign tumor of the lymph vessels (lymphangioma) that consists of large, dilated lymphatic channels. The nomenclature can be confusing and they can also be referred to as macrocystic lymphangiomas. They usually present at or soon after birth and can grow to massive proportions. These tumors may cause life-threatening compression of the airway. They may be injected with a sclerosing agent (OK432, alcohol) or surgically excised.

Pharyngitis

Pharyngitis describes any inflammation of the throat and is one of the most common infections in medicine. Pharyngitis can have many different causes, including infectious (viral is far more common than bacterial), traumatic, and caustic causes, laryngopharyngeal reflux, allergy, and smoking.

Common agents causing infectious pharyngitis

- Viral: adenovirus, rhinovirus, herpes simplex virus (ulcerations), coxsackievirus (herpangina or hand-foot-mouth disease), and Epstein–Barr virus (infectious mononucleosis)
- The most common bacteria are streptococci, pneumocci, and *H. influenzae*.
- *Corynebacterium diphtheria*, characterized by grayish exudates
- *Bordetella pertussis* results in pharyngitis with tracheobronchitis and causes whooping cough.
- *Neisseria gonorrhea is* often sexually transmitted. It may be associated with joint pain and meningitis.

Group A beta-hemolytic streptococcus pharyngitis

Group A beta-hemolytic streptococcus (GABHS) is one of the most common causes of bacterial pharyngitis and is associated with the development of rheumatic fever, scarlet fever, and glomerulonephritis. For this reason, group A streptococcus should be suspected and treated in all cases of acute severe pharyngitis.

- Testing includes GABHS rapid antigen test (70%–90% sensitive), throat culture, and antistreptolysin-O (ASO) antibody.
- Treat with antibiotics. Penicillin is still effective.

Rheumatic fever

Rheumatic fever (RF) is characterized by diffuse swelling and inflammation involving soft tissue, the heart, joints, and blood vessels. The process is incompletely understood and may be secondary to systemic release of inflammatory mediators or instigation of an autoimmune process by the strep antigen. This occurs more often in children from ages 5 to 15 years. The incidence of RF is approximately 3% in untreated strep pharyngitis. Although rarely seen today, RF used to be one of the leading causes of cardiac valve disease worldwide and is still a significant public health issue in developing countries.

The cell surface marker of the group A streptococcus is called the M-protein, which has been linked to the pathophysiology of RF, post-streptococcal glomerulonephritis, and scarlet fever.

Diagnosis is based on Jones Criteria: two major or one major + two minor criteria are required in addition to proven infection with group A streptococcus.

- Previous streptococcus infection as documented by positive culture or rapid antigen testing and/or elevation in streptococcal antibody test (ASO).

- Major criteria include carditis, Aschoff bodies (subcutaneous nodules), erythema marginatum, migratory polyarthritis, and Sydenham's chorea.
- Minor criteria include arthralgia, fever, elevated acute-phase reactants on serology, and prolonged PR interval on electrocardiogram (EKG).

Scarlet fever

Scarlet fever is characterized by diffuse swelling and inflammation involving soft tissue, skin, and mucosa secondary to bacterial exotoxins. These exotoxins enable the spread of infection and are responsible for most of the local and systemic toxicity of these organisms. Pyrogenic or erythrogenic exotoxins are components linked to the development of the rash associated with scarlet fever.

- Signs and symptoms inlcude skin erythema (scarlet) and strawberry tongue.
- Dick test involves the intradermal injection of isolated erythogenic toxin. Susceptible individuals produce a local wheal and flare reaction.

Post streptococcal glomerulonephritis

Glomerulonephritis occurs about 7–14 days after the initial infection. Most cases occur after strep pharyngitis but can also occur after skin infections such as impetigo. It is thought to be the result of immune-complex deposition within the kidney or the stimulation of autoantibodies.

- Signs and symptoms include gross hematuria, generalized edema, mild hypertension, flank pain, oligouria, and retinal hemorrhages. It can lead to chronic kidney failure.
- Urinalysis shows red blood cells (RBC) and RBC casts.
- Treatment is supportive and most patients make a full functional recovery.

Tonsillitis

Tonsillitis, or infection of the tonsils, is commonly seen in ENT and general practice. Common bacterial pathogens are B-hemolytic streptococcus, moraxella, catarrhalis, and *Hemophilus influenzae*. Sometimes this occurs following an initial viral infection. Treatment consists of appropriate antibiotics, regular simple analgesia, oral fluids, and bed rest.

Signs of acute tonsillitis

- Sore throat
- Enlargement of the tonsils
- Exudate on the tonsils
- Difficulty swallowing
- Fever
- Malaise
- Halitosis
- Ear pain
- Trismus

Complications of tonsillitis

Airway obstruction This is very rare, but may occur in tonsillitis due to mononucleosis. The patient may experience severe snoring and acute sleep apnea. This may require rapid intervention, e.g., insertion of naso-pharyngeal airway or intubation.

Quinsy (peritonsillar abscess) This appears as a swelling of the soft palate and tissues lateral to the tonsil, with displacement of the uvula towards the opposite side. The patient is usually toxic with fever, trismus, and drooling. Needle aspiration or incision and drainage is required, along with antibiotics, which are usually administered intravenously.

Parapharyngeal abscess This is a serious complication of tonsillitis and usually presents as a diffuse swelling in the neck. Other deep neck space infections are also possible with tonsillitis, either from extension from the peritonsillar space or via suppurative lymphadenitis. Admission is required and surgical drainage is often necessary via an external neck incision.

Management

Patients with complicated tonsillitis and those who are unable to take enough fluid orally will need to be admitted to the hospital for rehydra-tion, analgesia, and intravenous antibiotics. Ampicillin should be avoided if there is any question of mononucleosis, because of the florid skin rash which will occur.

Infectious mononucleosis

Infectious mononucleosis ("mono") is also known as glandular fever or Epstein–Barr virus infection. It is common in teenagers and young adults. Patients with mono may present a similar picture to that of patients with acute bacterial tonsillitis, but with a slightly longer history of symptoms. Diagnosis relies on a positive monospot or Paul–Bunnell blood test (heterophil antibodies in serum), although early in the course of the disease this test can still show up negative.

Signs and symptoms
- Sore throat
- Fever
- Cervical lymphadenopathy
- White slough on tonsils
- Petechial hemorrhages on the palate
- Marked widespread lymphadenopathy
- Hepatosplenomegaly

Treatment
This is a self-limiting condition and treatment is largely supportive with painkillers, although patients may appreciate a short course of corticosteroids to decrease swelling. Intravenous (IV) fluids may be necessary if they cannot drink enough.

Complications
Patients should be advised to refrain from contact sports for 6 weeks because of the risk of a ruptured spleen, which can lead to life-threatening internal bleeding. Ampicillin is associated with a rash and should be avoided. Rarely, hemolytic anemia may be severe.

Tonsillectomy

This is one of the most commonly performed operations.

Indications for tonsillectomy

- Suspected malignancy in the presence of asymmetric tonsil or unusual-appearing tonsil (absolute indication)
- Children with obstructive sleep apnea (OSA) and/or cor pulmonale (absolute indication)
- As part of another procedure, such as ulvulopalatoplasty (UPP) for snoring
- Recurrent acute tonsillitis
- Three attacks per year for 3 years or
- Five attacks in any one year
- More than one quinsy

Big tonsils that are asymptomatic need not be removed. Removing the tonsils does not always prevent tonsillitis; remember the adenoids and lingual tonsils. It also does not prevent pharyngitis.

There are numerous methods for the removal of tonsils. Complete tonsillectomy involves dissecting the tonsils off the muscles of the fossa. Subcapsular tonsillectomy removes and debulks the tonsillar tissue, preserving the surrounding capsule. This technique has been used for obstructive sleep symptoms without significant infections.

Postoperative

Tonsillectomy is very painful. Patients should be advised that referred pain to the ear is common. Until the tonsillar fossa are completely healed, eating is very uncomfortable. Generally a soft diet is recommended postoperatively. Narcotics are generally needed.

In the immediate postoperative period, the tonsillar fossa becomes coated with a white exudate, which can be mistaken as a sign of infection.

Complications

Postoperative hemorrhage is a serious complication and occurs in approximately 2%–4% of cases.

- **Immediate postoperative hemorrhage** can occur in the first few hours after the operation; this will frequently necessitate a return trip to the operating room. This may be secondary to incomplete hemostasis, rupture of a vessel, release of a vasospastic artery, or hypertension.
- **A secondary hemorrhage** can occur any time within 2 weeks of the operation. It occurs because of neoangiogenesis within the wound bed. See Chapter 20, p. 424.
- The combination of postoperative nausea, vomiting, and dehydration is one of the most common reasons for hospital admission. Treatment is with pain control and IV fluids.

- Postoperative flash pulmonary edema is a rare but frightening condition in which the lungs fill up rapidly with fluid. This occurs as a response to the sudden decrease in airway pressure after relieving obstruction. It has been reported after tonsillectomy as well as after sleep apnea surgery. Treatment includes diuresis and intubation with the goals of increasing the pulmonary back pressure.
- *Eagle's syndrome* is a condition described as occurring after tonsillectomy. The hallmarks are persistent ear and throat pain with evidence of reactive calcification and fibrosis of the stylohyoid ligament or an elongated styloid process. Palpation of the tonsillar fossa should reproduce the pain. Diagnosis must be done very carefully and other disorders must be ruled out. Surgical treatment with removal of the styloid process and ligament has been used as treatment.

Tonsillar tumors

Benign tumors of the tonsils are very rare. But tonsillar stones (tonsiliths) with surrounding ulceration, mucus retention cysts, herpes simplex, or giant aphthous ulcers may mimic the more common malignant tumors of the tonsil.

Squamous cell carcinoma (SCC)

This is the most common tumor of the tonsil and is staged as oropharyngeal cancers in the AJCC guidelines. The other subsites within the oropharynx include the soft palate, base of tongue, and the lateral and posterior pharyngeal walls. Except for the posterior pharyngeal wall, there is a rich lymphatic drainage network from these areas and an early propensity for lymphatic involvement. Tonsillar SCC tends to occur in middle-aged and elderly people, but in recent years tonsillar SCC has become more frequent in patients under the age of 40. Many of these patients are also unusual candidates for SCC because they are nonsmokers and nondrinkers.

Signs and symptoms
- Pain in the throat
- Referred otalgia
- Ulcer on the tonsil
- Lump in the neck.

As the tumor grows it may affect the patient's ability to swallow and it may lead to an alteration in the voice—this is known as "hot potato speech."

Diagnosis is usually confirmed with a biopsy taken at the time of the staging panendoscopy. Fine-needle aspiration of any neck mass is also necessary. Imaging usually entails CT, MRI, and/or PET scan. It is important to exclude any synchronous head and neck or pulmonary tumor as well as metastatic disease with a chest X-ray and/or a chest CT scan.

Treatment
Treatment and management are dependent on the tumor size, lymph node spread, and distant metastasis.

Treatment options include the following:
- Radiotherapy alone
- Chemoradiotherapy
- Transoral laser surgery
- En-bloc surgical excision—this removes the primary and the affected nodes from the neck. Oropharyngeal cancers can be difficult to expose and often involve transfacial or transmandibular approaches. Robotic surgery may be making advancements in resection.
- Often it will be necessary to reconstruct the surgical defect to allow for adequate speech and swallowing afterward. Reconstructing the oropharyx and palate is difficult, and residual dysfunction is not uncommon. Reconstruction can vary from free tissue transfer, such as a radial forearm free flap, to the manufacture of a prosthetic or obturator.

Lymphoma

This is the second most common tonsil tumor.

Signs and symptoms

- Enlargement of one of the tonsils
- Lymphadenopathy in the neck—may be large
- Mucosal ulceration—less common than in SCC

Investigations

Fine-needle aspiration cytology may suggest lymphoma, but it rarely confirms the diagnosis. The specimens should be sent with a cell block in normal saline so that flow cytometry may be performed. A sample with cell architecture may be taken in an easily accessible lymph node with a true-cut or core biopsy needle used for liver biopsy. However, it is often necessary to perform an excision biopsy of one of the nodes. Because neck dissection is the standard protocol for removing SCC, excisional biopsy of an unexpected SCC can produce a problem associated with potentially seeding the neck with cancer and disrupting the normal system of lymphatic drainage.

Staging is necessary with imaging of the neck, chest, abdomen, and pelvis. Further surgical intervention is not required other than to secure a threatened airway.

Treatment

This usually consists of chemotherapy and/or radiotherapy.

Adenoidal enlargement

The *adenoid* is a collection of loose lymphoid tissue found in the space at the back of the nose. The eustachian tubes open immediately lateral to the adenoids. Enlargement of the adenoids is very common, especially in children. It may happen as a result of repeated upper respiratory tract infections (URTIs), which occur in children because of their poorly developed immune systems.

Signs and symptoms
- Nasal obstruction and congestion
- Nasal quality to the voice
- Mouth breathing, which may interfere with eating
- Rhinorrhea
- Snoring
- Obstructive sleep apnea syndrome (OSAS)
- Blockage of the eustachian tube with recurrent or chronic otitis media.

A diagnosis of adenoidal enlargement is usually suspected from the history. Use of a mirror or an endoscopic nasal examination will confirm the diagnosis.

The glue ear that arises as a result of poor eustachian tube function may cause hearing impairment. Adenoiditis, or infection of the adenoid, may allow ascending infections to reach the middle ear via the eustachian tube.

Treatment
An adenoidectomy is performed under a general anesthetic. The adenoids are usually removed using suction diathermy or curettage.

Complications
Hemorrhage (primary, reactionary, and secondary) This is a serious complication of an adenoidectomy, but is less common than with a tonsillectomy.

Velopharyngeal insufficiency (VPI) and nasal regurgitation The soft palate acts as a flap valve and separates the nasal and the oral cavity. If the adenoid is removed in patients who have even a minor palatal abnormality, it can have major effects on speech and swallowing. Velopharyngeal incompetence can occur in these patients, resulting in nasal regurgitation of liquids and air escape during speech. Patients with a cleft palate, bifid uvula, or submucosal palatal cleft are at high risk for developing this complication. Assessment of the palate should form part of the routine ENT examination before such an operation.

Obstructive sleep apnea

Obstructive sleep apnea (OSA) is a major public health problem and results in neurocognitive problems (poor productivity and accidents) as well as cardiovascular and pulmonary complications. Snoring and OSA are associated but distinct entities. Snoring is very commonly observed, whereas OSA is associated with specific findings on sleep study as well as clinical features of sleep deprivation. OSA affects approximately 1%–4% of middle-aged men. In children, upper airway resistance syndrome (UARS) is similar to OSA and is generally associated with adenotonsillar hypertrophy. In adults, OSA can be the result of narrowing anywhere in the upper respiratory tract.

Sleep apnea

- Obstructive sleep apnea: problem breathing during sleep secondary to anatomic obstruction of the upper airway. This is a much more common entity than central sleep apnea. Usually there is anatomic narrowing of the upper airway, which is further narrowed when supine and when the muscles of the pharynx and oral cavity are relaxed, resulting in reduced patency of the airway against the negative pressure created during inspiration.
- Central sleep apnea: problem with the breathing drive centers, often in the brainstem. This is not usually associated with the physical findings of OSA. It occurs more often in infants and in the elderly.

Signs and symptoms

- Snoring
- Apneas and hypopneas (see below)
- Arousals—nighttime awakenings, often gasping for breath
- Daytime somnolence
- Poor sleep and insomnia
- Morning headaches

Sleep study

A sleep study measures multiple components of sleep, including electro-encephalography (EEG) activity, EMG, leg movements, airflow monitor of respiration, EKG, oxygen saturation, and snoring sounds. The following definitions and indices are used:

- *Apnea* is cessation of breathing and airflow for at least 10 seconds.
- *Hypopnea* is reduced ventilation of at least 50% for at least 10 seconds, followed by an arousal and/or drop in oxygen saturation.
- Apnea-Hypopnea Index (AHI) = Apnea per hour + Hypopnea per hour. An AHI greater than 10 is considered abnormal.
- Respiratory effort-related arousal (RERA)
- Respiratory disturbance index (RDI) = Apnea per hour + Hypopnea per hour + RERA per hour. RDI greater than 15 is considered abnormal.

Complications and natural history

- Chronic sleep deprivation has been associated with motor vehicle accidents, poor job performance, and mood alterations.
- Cardiac conditions associated with OSA include hypertension, cardiovascular disease, myocardial infarction, and stroke.
- Pulmonary complications include pulmonary hypertension and cor pulmonale.

Medical treatments

Treatment should be geared toward treating any medical comorbidities, weight loss, and any respiratory issues such as asthma, emphysema, and nasal congestion or allergies.

- Behavioral treatment includes weight reduction, avoidance of respiratory depressants such as alcohol for sleep, positional changes during sleep (avoiding supine position), and head elevation. A 10% reduction in weight is associated with a 25% improvement in AHI. Avoiding airway irritants such as smoking and controlling allergies are also helpful.
- Continuous positive airway pressure (CPAP) is the most reliable treatment for OSA. The CPAP machine is essentially an air compressor and blower that delivers a constant pressure to the airway. This "pneumatic splint" helps maintain airway patency. The patient is required to wear a tight-fitting mask over the nose and or mouth at night. The major obstacle to therapy is patient compliance, which is reported to be approximately 60%.
- Oral splints are intraoral devices that can help a select group of patients maintain airway patency. The splints generally work by helping advance the mandible forward and increasing the distance between the posterior pharyngeal wall and the base of tongue.

Surgery for obstructive sleep apnea

The success of surgical treatment for OSA has been variable. Although short-term results of most procedures are successful, long-term reduction and improvement in AHI or RDI are less impressive. Because of the variability in anatomy and the multiple sites of potential airway blockage, a single operation or approach is difficult to apply. There are some surgeries with high success at treating snoring but variable success for OSA.

- Uvulapharyngopalatoplasty (UPPP) involves removing the uvula, tonsils, faucial arches, and a portion of the soft palate and advancing the soft palate forward. It is the most common surgery for OSA, with a reported success rate of approximately 50%.
- Palatoplasty has been performed in a variety of ways. Laser, sclerosing agents, implantable pillars, radiofrequency waves, and coblation have been used to alter and stiffen the palate to reduce airway obstruction and snoring.

- Mandibular and maxillary advancement involves controlled osteotomies to enlarge the pharyngeal airway. The reported success rate has been approximately 90%, but the procedure is associated with significant morbidity.
- Tracheotomy has been performed for severe OSA and is considered a surgical option. Results are very good; however, symptoms must be severe, and very few patients are willing to undergo this procedure.

The nose and sinuses

Structure and function of the nose

Structure

The structure of the nose is made up of four parts:

- The surface anatomy—see Fig. 6.1 for the surface landmarks.
- The nasal skeleton—composed of the two nasal bones, the paired upper lateral and lower lateral alar cartilages, and the nasal septum, covered in subcutaneous tissue and skin (see Fig. 6.2).
- The internal anatomy, which includes the septum of the nose, which forms the medial wall of the nasal cavity. The septum is composed of a quadrangular-shaped cartilage anterior and a portion of the ethmoid bone called the perpendicular plate posterior. The septum articulates onto the floor of the nose on the vomer bone. There are four pairs of bony turbinates on the lateral wall. Also called concha (the Latin term for scroll, see Fig. 6.3), these structures serve to direct air posterior, reduce turbulence, and increase surface area contact for the mucosa. Each turbinate encloses a space termed the meatus. Various outlets for the paranasal sinuses and nasolacrimal duct flow into these meatal spaces.
- The osteomeatal complex (OMC) (Fig. 6.4) is a region within the middle meatus that forms the outflow tracts of the maxillary, frontal, and ethmoid sinuses. This is a key functional area of the nose under-neath the middle turbinate. Understanding the anatomy of the OMC is essential to understanding the etiology of sinus disease (see Fig. 6.5).

Knowing the anatomical terms for parts of the nose helps you to describe the site of lesions accurately as well as document the findings of examinations accurately.

Function

The nose is the main route for inspired air, and its structure is related to this function. As the air passes over the large surface area of the turbinates, the inspired gases are warmed and humidified. Mucus on the mucosa of the nose removes large dust particles from the air. The nasal cavity allows for chemicals and odorants to stimulate the olfactory neuroepithelium at the region of the cribriform plate.

The voice resonates in the sinuses and nose, and this provides character to the speech. Patients with very obstructed nasal passages have what is often described as a nasal quality to their speech.

Pneumatization of the sinuses, which are air-filled spaces, reduces the weight of the skull and may also have developed as a crumple zone to protect the brain from injury.

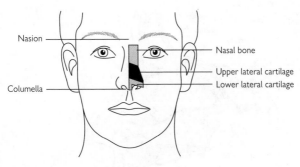

Fig. 6.1 Diagram of the surface markings of the nose.

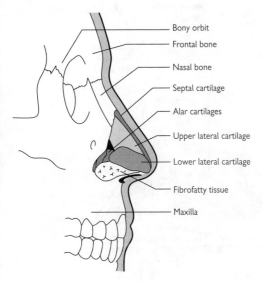

Fig. 6.2 Diagram of the nasal skeleton.

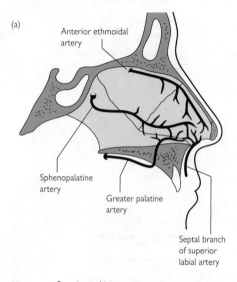

(a)

Anterior ethmoidal artery

Sphenopalatine artery

Greater palatine artery

Septal branch of superior labial artery

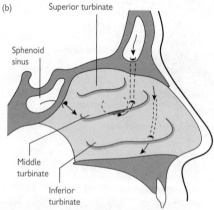

(b)

Superior turbinate

Sphenoid sinus

Middle turbinate

Inferior turbinate

Fig. 6.3 Diagram of the internal structure of the nose.

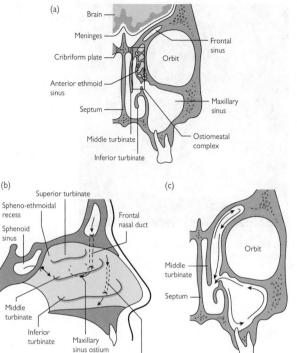

Fig. 6.4 The osteomeatal complex.

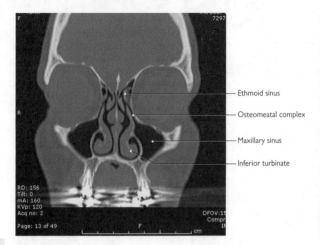

Ethmoid sinus

Osteomeatal complex

Maxillary sinus

Inferior turbinate

Fig. 6.5 Non-contrast coronal CT scan of the paranasal sinuses showing osteomeatal unit.

Rhinitis

Rhinitis is an inflammation of the nasal lining. Rhinitis may be diagnosed if a patient has two out of three of the following symptoms for more than 1 hour every day for over 2 weeks.

Symptoms

- Blocked nose and nasal congestion
- Rhinorrhea or running nose—including postnasal drip
- Sneezing

This condition is very common. Approximately one in six adults suffers from rhinitis.

Causes

There are a multitude of factors that cause rhinitis. It may be caused by several different factors, so it is important to treat each different cause. The symptoms of rhinitis may also be part of systemic disease (see Table 6.1).

The most common forms of rhinitis are allergic and infective. Classification of the disease is shown in Table 6.1.

History

It is important to take a full history to determine the cause of rhinitis. History of atopy or asthma, and any seasonal variation in the symptoms are relevant to diagnosis. Documenting the main symptoms—blockage, running, and sneezing—and noting which one is predominant will help in treatment selection.

The patients should be asked what medications are being used and about their smoking history—almost every smoker has a degree of rhinitis. The patient should be asked about any previous treatment for rhinitis, including its duration and effectiveness.

Investigations

- *Anterior rhinoscopy*—used to look for enlarged swollen turbinates (a blue tinge often indicates an allergic rhinitis) or nasal polyps.
- *Rigid nasal endoscopy*—used to examine the middle meatus for mucopus, polyps, and patency of the ostia.
- *Skin allergy tests*—performed for the testing of environmental allergies. Several different forms of the test are available. All involve the placement of tiny amounts of test substances on the skin. For skin prick and intradermal testing, a pin prick is made—a positive result leads to a small raised, red, itchy patch, which can be quantified. These tests are very sensitive and specific, and skin testing can be used as basis for immunomodulation therapy.
- *Radioallergosorbent test (RAST)*—a blood test that measures IgE levels to various substrates.
- *Peak flow*—there is a high degree of association between rhinitis and asthma. Peak flow measures the amount of airflow that can be generated during forced expulsion of air. Peak flows are reduced with asthma and are measured with pulmonary function testing.

Table 6.1 Classification of rhinitis

Common			Rare
Allergic	Infections	Other	Part of systemic disease
Seasonal	Acute	Idiopathic	Primary mucus defect
Perennial	Chronic	NARES (non-allergic rhinitis with eosinophilia)	• Cystic fibrosis
			• Young's disease
		Drug-induced	Primary ciliary dyskinesis
		Beta-blockers	• Kartagener's syndrome
		Oral contraceptives	Immunological
		Aspirin	• SLE
		NSAIDS	• Rheumatoid arthritis
		Local decongestants	AIDS
		Autonomic/vasomotor	Antibody deficiency
		Atrophic	Granulomatous disease
		Neoplastic	• Wegener's/sarcoidosis
			Hormonal
			• Hypothyroidism
			• Pregnancy

Medical treatment of rhinitis

Treatment of rhinitis is related to the underlying etiology of the condition.

Allergen avoidance

If the patient's rhinitis is caused by an allergy, skin prick testing can identify allergens to be avoided. It gives visual feedback to the patient to confirm the diagnosis. Following a positive skin prick test, allergen-avoidance information can be given.

Pharmacological treatments

Each of the different medications has different effects on symptoms (see Table 6.2).

- Steroids should ideally be delivered topically to the nasal mucosa as sprays or drops. When using drops, it is important to administer in the correct position, i.e., head down. Oral steroids can be very effective, but their systemic effects limit their long-term use.
- Antihistamines—non-sedating antihistamines are effective against sneezing, itching, and watery rhinorrhea. Used systemically they can be effective for other atopic problems such as watery eyes. They are not useful for symptoms of blockage.
- Topical nasal decongestants such as neosynephrine and oxymetazolone are only useful in the short term at the start of other therapy or for flying. Prolonged use can produce intractable rhinorrhea of rhinitis medicamentosa secondary to chronic vasoconstriction.
- Systemic decongestants such as phenylephrine or pseudoephedrine are useful in short courses but can elevate blood pressure and have sympathetic side effects.
- Ipratropium bromide is an anticholinergic medication commonly used for asthma treatment. An intranasal preparation is effective for watery vasomotor type rhinitis.
- Sodium cromoglycate is a mast cell stabilizer that prevents the degranulation of mast cells and is useful for allergic rhinitis.

Table 6.2 Medications and their symptom control*

	Sneezing	Discharge	Blockage	Anosmia
Cromoglycate	++	+	+	–
Decongestant	–	–	+++	–
Antihistamine	+++	++	+/–	–
Ipratropium	–	++	–	–
Topical steroids	+++	++	++	+
Oral steroids	++	++	+++	++

* Degree of benefit where +++ is maximum and – is minimum.

Surgical treatment of nasal obstruction

Rhinitis is considered a disease of the nasal mucosa, thus the role of surgery is limited. The primary goal of surgery is to improve nasal airflow and eliminate obstruction of sinus ostia. Surgery to improve nasal function may be a useful adjunct to other treatments. Even if a surgically correctable problem is found, it is worth a trial of medical therapy alone in the first instance as this often brings a high rate of symptom resolution. It is also worth obtaining a CT scan of the paranasal sinuses if surgery is considered, to review the need for sinus surgery.

Turbinate reduction

The turbinates often hypertrophy in all types of rhinitis, but particularly in allergic rhinitis. Their hypertrophy often obstructs the airway to such a degree that it is impossible to deliver topical medication. Reduction can be achieved by several means:

• Surface linear cautery—burning the surface
• Submucous diathermy—burning under the surface
• Cryotherapy—freezing
• Outfracture—lateralizing the turbinates out of the airway
• Submucosal conchopexy—changing the shape of the turbinate
• Trimming or excising the turbinate

Although these techniques are effective in improving the airway, additional medical therapy is often needed to prevent recurrence of the hypertrophied mucosa. The technique of turbinate excision has the potential for the development of atrophic rhinitis, a disabling condition marked by nasal congestion and the development of large obstructing crusts composed of inspissated nasal secretions.

Septal surgery

A deviated septum may need to be corrected to improve nasal function and help medication delivery. Techniques for septoplasty vary and include resection of the deviated portion of the septum.

Functional endoscopic sinus surgery

This surgery is aimed at the osteomeatal complex—its goal is to remove blockage in the critical area and restore the normal function and drainage of the sinuses. It could benefit patients with sinusitis who do not respond to medical treatments.

Recommended reading

Rosenfeld RM, Andes D, Bhattacharyya N, *et al.* (2007). Clinical practice guideline: Acute sinusitis. *Otolaryngol Head Neck Surg* **137**:S1–S31.

Olfaction

Olfactory physiology

Olfaction is a special sensory pathway and is the result of binding between environmental chemicals, the odorants, and olfactory receptor cells within the nasal cavity. The olfactory cleft is the region just below the cribriform plate. Neuroepithlial cells perforate the cribriform plate to gain exposure to the nasal cavity. The olfactory nerve is the collective central processes of the olfactory receptor cells. The region is notable because there is direct contact between neurons and the environment. The trigeminal nerve also participates in smell via sensory receptors in the nasal mucosa. These receptors primarily respond to chemical irritants and are mediated by neuropeptide P.

Olfactory dysfunction and loss of smell

Olfactory dysfunction can manifest itself in a variety of ways. *Anosmia* is the inability to smell, whereas *hyposmia* is a decreased smelling acuity. *Dysosmia* is disordered smell, usually of something unpleasant, and *phantosmia* is the sensation of odors that are not present.

Signs and symptoms Anosmia and hyposmia are the most frequent olfactory complaints and can be the result of disorders in the nasal cavity, mucosa, neurons, or central nervous system. Nasal causes are generally the result of mucosal abnormality and impaired respiration and delivery of odorants to the olfactory cleft. Examples include rhinitis of any form, smoking, nasal polyps, nasal septal deviation, and impaired mucociliary action. Damage to the olfactory epithelium can occur as the result of infection, head injury, cranial base surgery, or hemorrhage. Central nervous system disorders such as Parkinson disease and especially Alzheimer disease are associated with smelling dysfunction. Systemic disorders such as metabolic disorders (thiamine deficiency, hypothyroidism) and those from toxin exposure can also impair olfaction. Kallman's syndrome is a congenital disorder characterized by midline neural fusion defects and is characterized by anosmia in conjunction with an incomplete olfactory stalk or hypothalamus in addition to hypogonadism. Dysosmia and phantosmia may be the result of temporal lobe disorders such as seizure or depression.

Examination A careful and systemic evaluation of the nasal cavity and nasopharynx should be performed. Taste complaints are commonly associated with smelling symptoms and should be evaluated. Testing is based on suspected etiology, but an evaluation of the nasal cavity and sinuses should be made with endoscopy. A CT scan or MRI of the nose and skull base can be ordered to evaluate for presence of mucosal thickening at the cribriform plate or chronic sinusitis or skull base neoplasm. There are also objectives tests for smelling such as the University of Pennsylvania Smell Identification test.

Treatment Treatment depends on the etiology and whether reversible causes are addressed. For rhinitis and mucosal damage, nasal saline rinses and nasal steroids are first line. Although the neuroepithelium can regenerate, the process may take years.

Sinusitis

Sinusitis is inflammation of the sinuses. It is often considered a continuation of the spectrum of rhinitis and often occurs in conjunction with upper respiratory tract infections (URTIs).

The work of Messerklinger has shown that effective sinus drainage occurs through the osteomeatal complex (see Fig. 6.4, p. 113). The sinus mucosa is lined with respiratory epithelium, which is ciliated pseudostratified columnar epithelium. The mucous environment is stratified and composed of multiple layers. Mucociliary action directs the flow of this layer into the sinus outflow tracts at a rate of approximately 1 cm per second. The sinuses normally do not accumulate mucus. Obstruction of the osteomeatal complex due to anatomical or mucosal problems impairs sinus drainage and leads to obstructed outflow, which predispose to infection. This can occur as an acute phenomenon (see p. 123) or as a chronic condition (see p. 125). Recurrent attacks of sinusitis can create an environment of chronic hypoxia and ciliary stasis.

Depending on the location of the infection, symptoms can vary from facial pain and pressure to headaches and swelling. The four paired sinuses vary in frequency of involvement and sinusitis can afflict all of them or individually. The maxillary sinuses are the most frequently involved, followed by the ethmoids, frontals, and sphenoid sinuses.

Acute sinusitis

Acute sinusitis is defined as sinus inflammation of less than 4 weeks' duration. It is one of the most common reasons for ambulatory visits and is the fifth leading diagnosis for antibiotic use. It is caused by an acute bacterial or viral infection and often develops after a preceding upper respiratory tract infection.

Signs and symptoms
- Preceding upper respiratory infection
- Nasal obstruction and discharge
- Severe facial pain over the sinuses, particularly the maxilla/cheeks
- Pain that is worse on bending down or coughing.
- Tenderness over the sinuses

Investigations
- An anterior rhinoscopy to examine the inside of the nose
- A rigid nasal endoscopy often shows pus in middle meatus or edematous mucosa. The mucopus usually drains posteriorly and can be seen with the endoscope in the nasopharynx.
- The maxillary and frontal sinuses can be evaluated for absence of transillumination. Normally in a clear sinus, a light source pressed against the cheek (for maxillary) or the frontal (forehead) sinuses will illuminate the cavity. For maxillary sinuses, transillumination is often best seen in the mouth through the palate. If the sinus is filled with fluid, there is no transillumination.
- Imaging for acute sinusitis is not routine. Facial X-rays can show fluid-filled areas.

Treatment
In healthy adults, medication alone is usually effective.
- Antibiotics may be given if bacterial infection is suspected. Generally antibiotics are prescribed for symptoms greater than 7 days' duration or for very severe symptoms. The most common community-acquired pathogens are *Streptococcus. pneumoniae*, *Haemophilu influenza*, and *Moraxella catarrhalis*. Anaerobic organisms are rare but can be associated with dental problems associated with the upper teeth. The length of treatment is 7–10 days.
- Decongestant—oxymetolozine 0.5% nasal spray for 3–5 days only. Systemic decongestants such as phenylephrine or pseudoephrine and antihistamines can also be used.
- Saline nasal sprays several times per day or a netty pot to wash out nasal secretions and crust. Steroid nasal sprays such as fluticasone nasal spray can be administered for 2 weeks.
- If sinus symptoms do not resolve, consider a sinus washout or culture and a CT scan of the paranasal sinuses.

In immunocompromised patients, consider a sinus washout and culture to obtain microbiology for more effective antimicrobial treatment; do not forget to culture and stain for fungal elements. Patterns of antibiotic resistance vary from region to region.

Recurrent acute sinusitis

Patients presenting with a history of recurrent sinusitis are often difficult to diagnose because, in the absence of an acute infection, there may be no abnormal physical signs. Even CT scans may be entirely normal. If the history is good and the CT shows anatomic predisposition for outflow obstruction, then functional endoscopic sinus surgery (FESS) is appropriate if the number of episodes of infection is sufficient to cause disruption to the person's lifestyle.

Differential diagnosis of sinusitis

- Migraine—typical or nonclassical migraine symptoms may mimic sinus symptoms, as can other headache disorders.
- Dental problems
- Temporomandibular joint disorders
- Trigeminal neuralgia
- Neuralgias of uncertain origin
- Atypical facial pain

Remember that the CT paranasal sinuses may be normal unless the patient is symptomatic and diagnosis may be difficult to make. Consultations with neurology and oral surgery in a multidisciplinary setting for headache treatment are useful.

Chronic sinusitis

Chronic sinusitis is an inflammation of the sinuses that lasts more than 6 weeks. Diagnosing chronic sinusitis, like diagnosing acute sinusitis, may be difficult, as other causes of facial pain may mimic it.

Investigation for chronic sinusitis should include evaluation for systemic disorders. Diseases that affect ciliary function (Kartagener's syndrome), mucus secretions (Cystic fibrosis), and the immune system (HIV and diabetes) should be considered, especially if there are disproportionate symptoms or unusual organisms. These conditions are especially important because they may predispose to the potentially devastating complications of sinusitis.

Signs and symptoms
- Pressure in the face, which gets worse on bending over
- Pain when flying, particularly when descending
- A feeling of nasal obstruction—can be objective or subjective
- Rhinitis—runny or blocked nose and sneezing
- Anosmia or hyposmia
- Postnasal drip
- Cough (especially in pediatrics)
- Halitosis (also common in pediatrics)

Investigations
- Nasal examination is performed to check the patency of the airway and appearance of the nasal mucosa.
- Anterior rhinoscopy is used to examine the septum and nasal cavity.
- Nasal endoscopy is used to examine the middle meatus and look for nasal polyps. Attention should be directed at potential blockages of the sinus ostia. Anatomy such as nasal septal deviation, paradoxical curvature of the middle turbinate, lateralized uncinate process, hypertrophic turbinates, and concho bullosa may contribute to chronic sinusitis and are amenable to surgical treatment.
- CT scanning—a non-contrast CT scan of the paranasal sinuses may be very valuable (Fig. 6.5). The purpose is not necessarily to make the diagnosis of sinusitis but to examine the sinus outflow anatomy.

Treatment
Eighty percent of patients respond to medical therapy. This will involve one or more of the following medication for at least 3 months:
- Intranasal steroid for inflammation and edema of the mucosa
- Oral antihistamine such as cetirizine hydrochloride

If medical treatment fails, the following treatments may be considered:
- Allergy testing
- Prolonged course of antibiotics for greater than 3 weeks' duration. The organisms are similar to those found in acute sinusitis but also include more anaerobes, *S. aureus*, and *H. influenza*.
- Functional endoscopic sinus surgery—extent is dictated by disease process at surgery
- Septoplasty may be necessary in addition to above.

Pediatric sinusitis

Development of sinuses

- Maxillary sinus is the first to develop in utero and is present at birth. This is the most common site of sinusitis.
- Ethmoid sinuses are present at birth and expand to reach adult size by age 15 years. Involvement of the ethmoid sinuses can lead to orbital, cavernous sinus and CNS complications.
- Frontal sinuses do not appear until age 5–6 years and are frequently hypoplastic in adults.
- Sphenoid sinuses form from evagination of nasal mucosa into the sphenoid bone.

Signs and symptoms

The most common symptoms are nasal congestion, cough, and halitosis. Purulent nasal drainage may be present as well as fever. Predisposing risk factors in children include adenoid hypertrophy, extraesophageal reflux, and asthma. Congenital immunoglobulin deficiencies and Cystic fibrosis should be considered during workup.

Treatment

Treatment in children is similar to that in adults. The most common pathogens are streptococcus, *S. pneumonia*, *M catarrhalis,* and *H. influenza*. Surgery is generally not necessary.

Special considerations

Cystic fibrosis is an autosomal recessive disease that affects mucus production. The genetic defect is well characterized and involves a mutation in the CF transmembrane conductance regulator. The mutation alters the transportation of chlorine and water and affects exocrine function. The result is formation of thick tenacious mucus that is difficult to clear and creates a nidus for infection. Almost all patients with CF have sinusitis. Approximately 10% also have nasal polyps. There are associated problems with the bronchopulmonary system, pancreas, and hepatobiliary systems. Diagnosis is made on the basis of a sweat chloride test. Organisms frequently found causing sinusitis are *Pseudomonas aeruginosa*, *S. aureus*, *E. coli,* and fungus.

Kartagener's syndrome is a frequently tested but rarely seen congenital disorder of ciliary function. The mutation results in deficiency in the outer dynein arm and in primary ciliary dyskinesis. The clinical manifestations include recurrent sinusitis, otitis media, and male infertility. The classic Kartagener's triad is chronic sinusitis, bronchiectesis, and situs inversus (the heart is on the right side of the chest). Diagnosis is made on biopsy of the nasal mucosa with electron microscopic evaluation of the cilia. Sinus drainage becomes gravity dependent.

Complications of sinusitis

Mucociliary damage

Long-standing or chronic sinusitis can lead to mucociliary failure. This means that the sinus cannot drain properly, even if it is anatomically ventilated. Cigarette smoke will also paralyze cilia action, so smoking should be avoided by those with sinusitis. Patients develop chronic crusting and dryness and a sense of nasal congestion. Treatment is supportive with aggressive nasal hydration.

Orbital complications

The proximity of the sinuses, especially the ethmoids, to the orbit can result in concomitant infections. An unresolved episode of acute ethmoid or pansinusitis may lead to orbital complications as shown in Fig. 6.6. The pathways to spread are usually through a weakness in the lamina papyracea or via the communication between the ethmoid veins to the ophthalmic veins. Management of this problem is dealt with in the emergencies section in Chapter 20 (see p. 417). The Chandler classification of orbital complications is shown in Fig. 6.6. The infections generally follow a stepwise progression.

- Preseptal edema and cellulitis—inflammation is limited to the periorbital area. The orbital septum provides a barrier to spread of infection directly into the orbit. There is chemosis and periorbital swelling and fever but no vision changes.
- Postseptal edema and cellulitis—inflammation is posterior to the orbital septum and effects the orbit. This causes proptosis, diplopia with limitation of the extraocular muscles, chemosis, and vision changes.
- Subperiosteal abscess—a collection of pus forms between the bone and the periosteum. Requires surgical drainage. Signs include proptosis, diplopia, and vision changes.
- Interconal abscess—orbital abscess within the soft tissues of the orbit. Presents with proptosis, chemosis, diplopia, and blindness. Surgical drainage is required.
- Cavernous sinus thrombosis. See below.

Cavernous sinus thrombosis

Infection of the perinasal skin, sinuses, and nasal cavity can spread retrograde into the cavernous sinus because of a lack of valves in the ophthalmic venous system. This can result in septic embolic-causing infections, inflammation, and eventually thrombosis. The most common organism here is *S. aureus*. Clinical manifestations include spiking fevers (a "picket fence" pattern of fevers), diplopia, chemosis, and blindness. Treatment is with broad-spectrum IV antibiotics and drainage of involved sinuses. The role of anticoagulation and steroids is controversial.

Intracranial complications

Meningitis, epidural, subarachnoid, and brain abscesses can result from infections of the sinuses. The posterior lamina of the frontal sinuses is thin and is shared directly with the dura of the frontal lobe. The posterior lamina also has numerous perforations made by diplopiac veins that can expose the intracranial contents to infection. Spread of infection from the frontal sinuses can cause problems as shown in Fig. 6.7. Similarly, extension of infection from the ethmoids and sphenoid sinuses can cause meningitis at the skull base.

Pott puffy tumor

Ongoing frontal sinusitis can lead to osteomyelitis of the frontal bone. A soft, boggy swelling then appears on the skin of the forehead. Treatment is surgical debridement and parenteral antibiotics. The disorder was given this colorful name by Sir Percival Pott, an English surgeon in the mid-1700s.

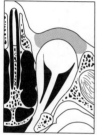
1. Preseptal edema

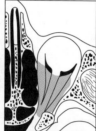
2. Postseptal edema

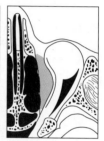
3. Subperiosteal abscess

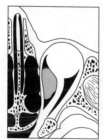
4. Interconal abscess

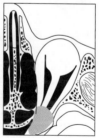
5. Cavernous sinus involvement

Fig. 6.6 Chandler classification of orbital complications.

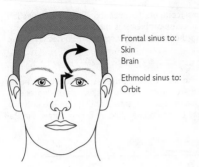

Frontal sinus to:
Skin
Brain

Ethmoid sinus to:
Orbit

Fig. 6.7 Pathways of spread for intracranial complications.

Fungal sinusitis

Fungal infections of the sinuses can manifest in different ways, from indolent chronic inflammation to rapidly fatal, invasive infections. Host immune response is the primary predictor for infection, and any sinus complaints in immunocompromised patients need to be taken seriously.

Fungal histology

Generally the identity of the fungal specimen is based on a culture or smear collected from the sinuses. Gomori silver stain is specific for fungal elements.

- Aspergillosis is septated and Y-shaped. Branches occur at 45° angles.
- Mucormycosis is non-septated with 90° branching hyphae.

Fungal ball (mycetoma)

This is a noninvasive form of fungal infection characterized by formation of a fungal collection within the sinuses. A CT scan of the paranasal sinuses shows a very discrete heterogeneous mass with multiple calcifications. Treatment is with surgical debridement.

Allergic fungal sinusitis

This is considered an immune response to colonized fungus rather than a true infection. There is usually a history of atopy, and signs and symptoms are similar to those of allergic rhinitis and chronic sinusitis. There is mucosal thickening along with polyps. On biopsy, there are fungal elements present with allergic mucin and nasal eosinophilia.

Chronic invasive fungal sinusitis

This is a more indolent form of fungal infection with invasion of the soft tissues. The symptoms are suggestive of chronic sinusitis, but there may be evidence of local invasion to adjacent structures. Biopsy shows invasive fungal elements and treatment is surgical debridement with long-term intravenous antifungals.

Invasive fungal sinusitis

This is considered an acute sinus emergency. Invasive fungal sinusitis is usually caused by Aspergillosis or Mucor and occurs almost exclusively in immunocompromised patients. Patients with HIV or diabetes and those undergoing chemotherapy or bone marrow transplant are at highest risk. Mortality is 50%. This condition causes soft tissue necrosis in the nasal cavity, palate, and external nose. There may be little or no pain, as there is a predilection for early neural and vascular invasion. Management is based on early recognition and identification, with swift surgical debridement and IV antifungals.

Nasal polyps

Simple nasal polyps are part of the spectrum of rhinosinusitis as the lining of the nose becomes inflamed and thicker. These polyps are edematous sinus mucosa, which prolapse to fill the nasal cavity to a variable extent. They are common, and their cause is unknown.

Signs and symptoms
- Variable symptoms—with the season or with URTI
- Rhinitis—blocked or runny nose and sneezing
- Sinusitis—due to osteomeatal obstruction
- Nasal obstruction
- Appearance of the polyps at the anterior nares
- Proptosis when severe

Investigations
- Anterior rhinoscopy—inferior turbinates are often incorrectly diagnosed as polyps; a rhinoscopy can help avoid this misdiagnosis (see Fig. 6.8).
- Rigid nasal endoscopy
- CT scan to evaluate for sinus inflammation
- Polyp size can be graded (see Fig. 6.9).

Treatment
- For small nasal polyps treat with nasal steroids.
- For large nasal polyps treat with nasal steroids and consider oral steroids.

If medical treatment fails, the following treatments should be considered:
- Surgical removal for obstructive polyps—if the patient is sufficiently symptomatic
- FESS
- Postoperative intranasal steroids
- Recurrences are common.

Samter's triad
This is the association of
- Aspirin sensitivity, making patients wheezy when they take aspirin
- Late-onset asthma
- Nasal polyps

It is caused by a defect in leukotriene metabolism. Polyps in this condition are florid and recur frequently.

Treatment
- Diet—refer patient to a dietician for advice on a low-salicylate diet. This is very bland and difficult to maintain.
- Intranasal steroids
- Repeat surgery as for nasal polyps above—the microdebrider is the atraumatic instrument of choice.
- Leukotriene antagonists, e.g., Monteleukast, to reduce the polyps—results may vary.

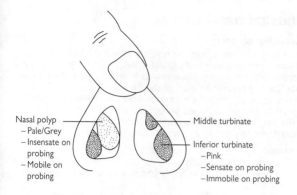

Fig. 6.8 Diagram of nasal polyp showing features compared with inferior turbinate.

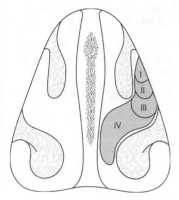

Fig. 6.9 Polyp size can be graded.

Unusual nasal polyps

Antrochoanal polyps

These polyps originate from the maxillary sinus and often present as a unilateral pendulous mass in the nasopharynx (see Fig. 6.10). The uncinate process directs the polyp posteriorly as it emerges from the maxillary sinus. They are uncommon and their cause is not known.

Macroscopically, the polyp is formed from a nasal component similar in appearance to a common nasal polyp.

The maxillary antral component is a thin, fluid-filled cyst. A small fibrous band joins the two as it passes out of the sinus.

Treatment

- CT scan to confirm the diagnosis
- Endoscopic removal of the polyps from its point of attachment in the maxillary sinus
- Caldwell–Luc approach for recurrent problem—an open sinus operation accessing the sinus via a cut in the mouth under the top lip

Childhood polyps

Polyps presenting in childhood are very unusual. They are usually associated with an underlying mucociliary abnormality such as cystic fibrosis or Kartagener's syndrome.

Investigations

- Consider a chloride sweat test, the diagnostic test for cystic fibrosis.
- Send biopsy to check that it is not a tumor.
- Get a fresh sample of nasal lining for special tests of ciliary function.
- Get a sample for electron microscopy to check the cillary structure.

Treatments

- Medical treatment with steroids
- Surgical removal

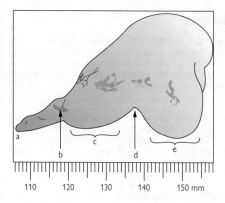

Fig. 6.10 Antrochoanal polyp and its anatomical relations.

a = maxillary sinus attachment; b = maxillary ostium; c = osteomeatal complex;
d = posterior choana; e = nasopharynx

Septal problems

The nasal septum provides an important mechanical support for the external nasal skeleton, dividing the nasal cavity into two compartments. Problems with the nasal septum can lead to both a cosmetic and functional disturbance of the nose. The nose may look bent to one side and/or the nasal airway may be restricted.

Septal deviation

The causes of septal deviation can be either congenital or traumatic. A traumatic septal deviation could be the result of a broken nose. Congenital septal deviation can occur after birth trauma to the nose or the differential growth of the nasal septum compared to the rest of the skull.

Almost all nasal septae are deviated to some extent. Most people do not experience any problem, but some find that their airway has become restricted. Acoustic rhinomanometry and computer flow modeling have shown that deviations at the area of the nasal valve cause the most functional impairment to airflow.

The internal nasal valve is the area bordered by the septum anterior edge of the inferior turbinate and caudal edge of the upper lateral cartilage. This area is situated about 1 cm posterior to the nares and is the narrowest segment of the nasal airway.

The external nasal valve is the area of the nasal vestibule formed by the nasal alar cartilage, columella, and nasal sill.

Change in the relative position of any of these structures causes a change in the cross-sectional area of the nasal valve and will result in nasal congestion.

Investigations
- Anterior rhinoscopy to exclude other problems, e.g., rhinitis
- Cottle's test to exclude alar collapse
- Nasal endoscopy to exclude sinusitis

Treatment
- Three months' trial of an intranasal steroid
- Surgery—septoplasty, or a submucous resection (SMR), is an operation on the nasal septum to improve nasal breathing. Treatment of the turbinates is common.

Septal perforation

Septal perforation results in disruption of nasal airflow with increased turbulence. Common reasons for septal perforation include the following:
- Trauma or accident
- Septal surgery
- Granulomatous disease—this must be excluded before treating perforation (see p. 138).
  - Wegener's granulomatosis
  - Sarcoidosis
  - TB
  - Syphilis
- Cocaine use

Signs and symptoms
- Chronic nasal congestion
- Whistling—if there is a small anterior perforation
- Epistaxis
- Crusting of the nose at the site of the perforation

Treatment
- Aggressive nasal hydration with nasal saline sprays
- Apply petrolatum to the edge of the perforation.
- Treat epistaxis expectantly.
- Septal button—this is a silastic prosthesis fitted into the hole in the septum. Only half of patients find it tolerable and continue using it long term.
- Surgical septal repair—the results of surgery are variable even in experienced hands.

Granulomatous conditions

These are an uncommon group of diseases that are classified together because of their histological appearance—they all form granulomas. Signs and symptoms are generally nasal congestion, bleeding, and the presence of irregular granulation within the upper aerodigestive tract. Diagnosis is based on biopsy and associated clinical features.

Signs and symptoms
- The patient may present with nasal granulomas as part of the generalized condition, e.g., sarcoid.
- Patients may have isolated nasal findings such as epistaxis, nasal congestion, septal perforation (posterior in syphilis), or crusting on the nasal septum.

Investigations
- CBC
- Urinalysis
- ESR
- Syphilis serology
- ANCA
- Chest X-ray
- Nasal biopsy

Wegener's granulomatosis
Wegener's granulomatosis is an autoimmune vasculitis affecting the small vessels. The primary sites of involvement are the upper airway, lungs, and kidneys.
- Key features are granulomatous inflammation of the nose, subglottis, lungs, and glomerulonephritis.
- Septal perforation is a very common manifestation.
- Diagnosis is based on cytoplasmic antineutrophil cytoplasmic antibody (c-ANCA) pattern of immunofluorescence, biopsy, and urinalysis showing red blood cells and casts.
- Renal disease may be rapidly progressive and potentially fatal.
- Treatment is with steroids and immunosuppressants.

Churg–Strauss syndrome
Churg–Strauss syndrome is a small-vessel vasculitis marked by peripheral eosinophilia, granulomas, and allergic features.
- Key features are asthma, peripheral eosinophilia, sinusitis, pulmonary infiltrates, neuropathy, and granulomatous inflammation of the nose.
- Diagnosis is based on soft tissue biopsy showing eosinophilic vasculitis.
- Treatment is with steroids and cyclophosphamide.

Sarcoidosis
Sarcoidosis is a systemic granulomatous inflammatory disease of unknown etiology. The primary site is the lungs, although the patient may present with nasal granulomas as part of the generalized condition.
- See Chapter 7.

Syphilis

Although rare today, syphilis was once the scourge of the developing world. The manifestations of syphilis are varied and occur in a characteristic pattern. The spirochete *Treponema pallidum* is the infecting agent and it is usually transmitted sexually. Its characteristics are as follows:

- The incubation period is 2–6 weeks.
- There is a primary lesion or painless ulcer (chancre) of the mucosal membrane with lymphadenopathy.
- Secondary bacteremia with widespread mucocutaneous lesions and lymphadenopathy can occur.
- The latent phase has few physical signs.
- The tertiary phase is marked by destructive mucocuteneous lesions. On the nose, these gummas are painless granulomatous destruction of the midline nose. Infection of the central nervous system, meninges, and aorta may also occur.
- Septal perforation is often posterior in syphilis.
- Diagnosis is based on clinical suspicion and serum testing and biopsy can help. Nontreponemal antigen testing such as VDRL and rapid plasma reagin (RPR) are sensitive but not specific. Fluorescent treponemal antibody absorption (FTA-ABS) is more specific and sensitive.
- Treatment is with antibiotics; penicillin G is highly effective.

Rhinoscleroma

A granulomatous inflammation of the internal and external nose, rhinoscleroma is the result of an indolent infection by *Klebsiella rhinoscleromatis*. The infection follows a specific pattern:

- A catarrhal stage with nonspecific rhinitis symptoms.
- A proliferative stage with formation of granulomas. Biopsy of granulomas show Mukulicz cells (foamy histiocytes containing the intracellular bacteria). Nasal polyps, epistaxis, and septal perforation may result.
- A cicatricial stage with progressive mucosal fibrosis.

Treatment is with long-term antibiotics. Tetracycline and fluoroquinolones are commonly used. The larynx and trachea may also be infected.

Rhinosporidiosis

Rhinosporidium seebri is a spore-forming fungus that can infect the nose and conjunctiva. The infection is endemic to Africa, Pakistan, and India and is spread with contaminated water.

- The granulomas form a friable, strawberry red, polypoid nasal lesion. Biopsy shows fungal sporangia and submucosal cysts.
- The lesions are treated with excision and cautery and systemic antifungal medications.

Sinonasal masses

Sinonasal malignancy is dealt with in Chapter 15.

Congenital nasal masses

Encephaloceles These are the reasons not to biopsy intranasal masses without prior imaging. Encephaloceles result from failure to close embryologic spaces enclosing the anterior neuropore. This produces communication through the frontal or nasal bones that can result in meninges and brain tissue herniating in the nasal cavity or external nose. Encephaloceles communicate with the CNS. Biopsy may result in infection and cerebrospinal fluid (CSF) leak. Encephaloceles can occur in other embryologic fusion planes such as the occiput, sphenoid sinuses, and ethmoid sinuses. *Furstenburg's sign* is enlargement of the mass during valsalva or compression of the jugular veins. Beware of any nasal mass that swells with straining or crying.

Gliomas and nasal dermoids are like encephaloceles without the communication with the CNS. They are trapped, separated remnants of glial tissue (gliomas) or dura (dermoids). They do not enlarge with straining. They may have a remnant fibrous stalk attachment to the meninges.

Thornwaldt's cyst and Rathke's pouch cysts are remnants of the notochord that persist in the nasopharynx. They are smooth, midline, and generally asymptomatic masses.

Inverting papilloma

An inverted papilloma is a mucosal neoplasm of the nasal cavity associated with infection by human papilloma virus. The most common location is the lateral nasal wall. The tissue proliferates and may cause localized symptoms with expansion and erosion of adjacent bony structures such as the orbit, and may predispose to infection. The appearance is very similar to that of nasal polyps but they occur unilaterally. There is a 10% risk of malignant degeneration, and when incompletely resected they will recur. Surgery with complete resection is the appropriate treatment. Classically, this is performed in an en-bloc manner with medial maxillectomy via a lateral rhinotomy or facial degloving approach. However, endoscopic sinus surgery is now being performed for select lesions with good results.

Histologically this condition is characterized by an endophytic growth pattern of the epithelium, forming the "inverted" papillary appearance.

Allergy and immunotherapy

Allergy testing and treatment for upper-airway reactivity is a rapidly expanding discipline of Otolaryngology. Although there are five major types of hypersensitivity reactions, the majority of allergic rhinitis and sinusitis cases are type 1, immunoglobulin E (IgE)-mediated reactions.

Type 1 hypersensitivity

Immunoglobulin E is produced by plasma cells during antigen reaction. The IgE antibody binds to mast cells and basophils, which are the primary cell mediators of allergic reactions. Mast cells degranulate when two adjacent IgE proteins cross-link on the surface. The products of degranulation are histamine, proteases, leukotrienes, and prostaglandins.

- Acute phase: The reaction of the products of degranulation produces inflammation of the mucosal tissues, resulting in nasal congestion and rhinorrhea. This occurs within 5 minutes of exposure to the antigen.
- Late phase: The result of secondary factors that are activated by leukotrienes and other products of the acute phase. These products recruit other inflammatory cells and eosinophils and propagate the inflammation.

Immunotherapy

The goal of immunotherapy is to desensitize the allergic response by exposing the body to low levels of antigen. Although the precise mechanism of action is unclear, it is believed that this level of exposure alters the balance between IgG and IgE.

- It is not first-line therapy, as the treatments are expensive and time consuming, require a high degree of patient compliance, and are potentially dangerous (can cause anaphylaxis).
- Indications include very severe symptoms, failure of medical therapy, and unavoidable allergens.
- RAST test results and skin testing are used to select the allergens for treatment.
- Dosing of the allergen depends on the level of sensitization. Highly sensitive allergens are exposed at very low levels. The allergen is injected intramuscularly or subcutaneously.
- The amount of allergen administered is gradually increased over time.
- Immunotherapy has the potential for allergy control and long-term remission.

The salivary glands

Structure and function of the salivary glands

There are three pairs of major salivary glands—the parotid, the submandibular, and the sublingual. In addition, there are a several hundred minor salivary glands scattered throughout the mucosa of the mouth and throat. They produce saliva that aids digestion and lubricates the food bolus.

The parotid gland

This gland lies on the side of the face, above the upper neck behind the angle of the mandible and in front of the ear. The gland is pyramid shaped and covered in thick fibrous tissue. The parotid duct, or *Stenson's duct,* opens into the mouth opposite the second upper molar tooth. The external carotid artery, retromandibular vein, and lymph nodes all lie within the parotid gland.

The facial nerve traverses the skull base and exits at the stylomastoid foramen. It then passes through the parotid gland as the pes anserinus, splitting into its five main divisions—temporal, zygomatic, buccal, mandibular, and cervical—as it does so. The facial nerve divides the parotid into a deep and superficial lobe.

The parotid gland and submandibular gland together account for almost 90% of total salivary flow. The parotid produces a more serous (watery) type of saliva and is highly activated during meals. The main cell type of the secretory unit is serous.

The submandibular gland

This gland lies just below the jaw in front of the angle of the mandible. The submandibular duct (Wharton's duct) runs from the deep lobe and ends as a papillae, at the front of the floor of the mouth (see Fig. 7.1). The duct usually exits lateral to the frenulum behind the incisors.

The lingual nerve, which gives sensation to the anterior two-thirds of the tongue, and the hypoglossal nerve, which provides the motor to muscles of the tongue, lie in close apposition to the deep surface of the gland.

The marginal mandibular branch of the facial nerve runs just deep to the platysma (subplatysmal plane) close under the skin that overlies the gland. Surgeons must be aware of these nerves to prevent iatrogenic damage.

A number of lymph nodes also lie close to or within the submandibular gland.

There are more mucinous glands within the submandibular gland than the parotid gland. Histologically, the gland is composed of a mix of serous and mucinous cells. The submandibular gland produces a mucinous saliva and has a higher basal flow rate than that of the parotid.

The sublingual gland

This is the smallest of the major salivary glands. It is found, or felt, in the floor of the mouth, running along the submandibular duct, into which it opens via 10–15 tiny ducts.

Parasympathetic nerve supply

See Fig. 7.2.

Parotid gland

The innervation signal originates from the inferior salivary nucleus of the medulla and is carried by the glossopharyngeal nerve to the otic ganglion via Jacobson's nerve. The fibers join the auriculotemporal nerve, which is a branch off of V3 to innervate the parotid gland.

Submandibular and sublingual gland

The innervation originates from the superior salivary nucleus within the pons and travels with the facial nerve via the nervus intermedius to the chorda tympani. The fibers join the lingual nerve off of V3 to innervate the submandibular and sublingual glands.

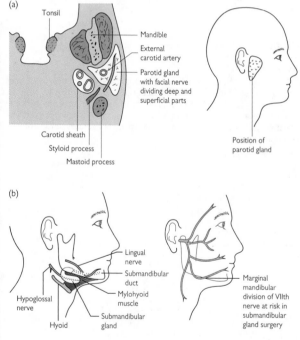

Fig. 7.1 Relation between parotid and submandibular glands.

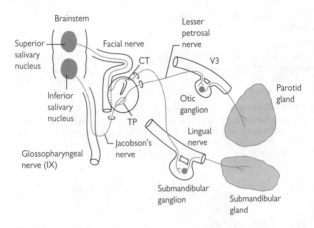

Fig. 7.2 Parasympathetic secretomotor nerve supply.

Salivary gland function

The secretory unit of the salivary glands is composed of acini cells and intercalated, striated, and excretory duct cells. Approximately 1.5 liters of saliva are produced daily. Saliva functions to lubricate food and hydrate mucosa, has immunoglobulins (IgA) with antibacterial properties, contains enzymes such as amylase to break down carbohydrates, and protects dental amalgam.

Disorders of salivation

Xerostomia

Xerostomia can occur with any condition that reduces salivary flow, such as radiation therapy, autoimmune processes such as Sjogren's disease, anticholinergic medications, and dehydration. Xerostomia seriously impacts quality of life and can compromise nutrition, oral hygiene, and hydration. The dryness can affect swallowing function and predispose to infection and bleeding. Treatment is generally supportive with aggressive hydration, pilocarpine, artificial saliva, and rigorous dental care.

Sialorrhea and ptyalism

Sialorrhea is excessive salivary production and is relatively rare compared to *ptyalism*, or loss of control of saliva with drooling. Hypersecretion of saliva can occur with certain medications and with infections of the gums and mouth. Drooling can occur in any condition that affects oral, facial, or laryngeal function. Common disorders causing ptyalism include Parkinsonism, stroke, oral incompetence, facial palsy, amyotrophic lateral sclerosis, and cerebral palsy. Constant drooling can result in problems with skin irritation or breakdown, oral infections, dental caries, electrolyte loss, and dehydration.

Treatment of ptyalism is geared toward the needs of the patient. Swallowing therapy can help with management of saliva and bolus preparation as can positioning of the head and neck during meals. Medications with anticholinergic effects are also effective but have systemic side effects. Scopalamine and glycopyrrolate are the most common agents. Surgical management includes removal of the submandibular glands, ligation or rerouting of the ducts, transection of Jacobson's nerve over the promontory of the tympanic plexus, and radiation therapy. Botulinum toxin injections into the glands are also used to temporarily chemodenervate the major salivary glands.

Salivary gland tumors

- 80% of all salivary gland tumors occur in the parotid gland.
- 80% of these are benign pleomorphic or mixed adenomas.
- 50% of submandibular gland tumors are malignant.
- 80% of minor salivary gland tumors are malignant.

Benign tumors

Pleomorphic adenomas or benign mixed tumor

Parotid pleomorphic adenomas are the most common salivary tumor. They are benign but have the potential for malignant transformation. They appear most often as an asymptomatic firm, mobile lump behind the angle of the mandible—this may displace the earlobe upward slightly. The tail of the parotid within the superficial lobe is the most common site. Weakness of the facial nerve suggests a malignant infiltration and the diagnosis must be questioned. Deep lobe parotid tumors can displace the oropharynx medially and may cause the tonsils to appear asymmetric. Deep lobe involvement occurs in approximately 10% of tumors.

Diagnosis is usually made via fine needle aspiration, and treatment is surgical. To prevent recurrence of adenomas, the surgeon should remove a cuff of normal parotid tissue around the lump and ensure that no tumor is spilt during excision. Commonly, this involves a superficial parotidectomy. The surgeon must take great care to identify and preserve the facial nerve during parotid surgery. Recurrent pleomorphic adenomas can present as multinodular masses that can recur within the wound bed or skin incision.

- Rare malignant transformation may occur to form carcinoma ex-pleomorphic adenoma.
- Even more rare is metastasizing mixed tumor, diagnosed by the presence of metastasis with benign histology.

Warthins tumor or papillary cystadenoma lymphomatosum

Warthin's tumor is the next most common benign tumor of the salivary glands. It most commonly affects elderly men. It occurs most often in the parotid gland, often in its tail—the part of the parotid that extends into the neck. This is the only tumor recognized as occurring bilaterally (occurs in 10%), and its cause is unknown. Unlike pleomorphic adenomas, which are firm, Warthin's tumors are usually soft, cystic, and compressible. Malignant transformation is rare. Fine-needle aspiration often reveals a cystic, fluid-filled mass with oncocytes (mitochondrial-rich cells) and lymphocytes. Technitium 99 scanning, which is concentrated by the mitochondria, can assist in the diagnosis. Treatment is surgical.

Oncocytomas

Oncocytomas are benign salivary gland tumors that are composed of exclusively of oncocytes. Oncocytes are present in numerous glandular tissues such as salivary glands and thyroid gland. Like Warthin's tumors, these tumors accumulate Technitium 99 which can aid in diagnosis. Treament is surgery.

Other benign salivary gland neoplasms
- Monomorphic adenoma
- Lipoma
- Cysts
- Hemangiomas

Pediatric salivary gland masses

Hemangiomas and pleomorphic adenomas are the most common benign salivary gland neoplasms occurring in children.

Hemangiomas

Hemangiomas are benign tumors of endothelial cell origin and represent one of the most common benign neoplasms in children. Although not made of salivary tissue, they represent almost 90% of all salivary gland tumors in children less than 1 year of age. They affect primarily the parotid gland and present as soft, compressible, painless, reddish masses. They go through a characteristic natural history marked by an early, rapidly proliferating growth phase followed by slow regression with soft-tissue fibrosis. Because spontaneous regression is the norm, treatment usually is supportive; however, surgery is considered for functional or cosmetic compromise.

Malignant tumors

Malignant salivary gland tumors are much less common than benign ones, but the symptoms can be similar—usually a lump in the neck. The following symptoms may suggest a malignant tumor:
- Pain
- Facial or other nerve weakness
- Skin involvement such as ulceration or fixation of the overlying skin
- Blood-stained discharge into the mouth
- Local lymph node enlargement suggests metastasis.

There are minor salivary glands in the mucosa of the nose, mouth, and throat. Neoplastic transformation here is often malignant.

Mucoepidermoid carcinomas

These are unusual tumors in that they have a range of aggressiveness from low to high. High-grade tumors require excision and postoperative radiotherapy, whereas low-grade tumors are generally treated with surgery alone.
- This is the most common salivary gland malignancy.
- The tumors are histologically composed of mucinous and epidermoid components.
- They are associated with radiation exposure.
- Differentiation between low-grade and high-grade lesions is based on percentage of mucinous elements. Low-grade lesions have a *higher* percentage of mucinous component.

Adenoid cystic carcinoma

These are the second most common malignant salivary gland tumors. They are slow growing and have a strong tendency to spread along the nerves. This perineural infiltration occurs early and is one reason for the poor long-term control rate of this disease. They can spread several centimeters beyond the palpable lump in this way. Treatment is with wide local excision of the tumor and postoperative radiotherapy.

The short-term or 5-year prognosis tends to be good, and patients with a recurrent tumor and even lung metastases may live for years. But the long-term or 25-year prognosis is poor, and in most cases patients will eventually die of this disease.

- It is the most common submandibular malignancy.
- Facial or other nerve weakness occurs early.
- Histologically it has a classical "Swiss cheese" appearance with a cribriform. High-grade lesions are composed of more solid sheets of cells.

Other salivary gland malignancies
- Acinic cell carcinoma
- Malignant mixed tumors
- Carcinoma ex-pleomorphic adenoma
- Metastasizing mixed tumor
- Carcinosarcoma
- Squamous cell carcinoma
- Lymphoma
- Adenocarcinoma
- Clear cell carcinoma
- Malignant oncocytoma
- Salivary duct carcinoma
- Undifferentiated carcinoma

Sialadenitis

Sialadenitis describes any inflammation of the salivary glands. Acute sialoadenitis is commonly the result of an acute infection of the submandibular or parotid gland. Suppurative sialoadenitis usually occurs in elderly or debilitated patients, who may be dehydrated and have poor oral hygiene. The most common organism of suppurative sialoadenitis is *Staphylococcus aureus*. The presence of calculi, or stones, within the gland may increase the risk of infection. Drugs such as the oral contraceptive pill, thiouracil, alcohol, and many others with anticholinergic activity may cause sialadenitis. Viral sialoadenitis is also very common, and mumps parotitis is one of the most common forms.

Chronic sialoadenitis may be the result of multiple infections with compromise of the outflow system, resulting in decreased flow and mucous plugs. There is fibrosis of the gland as well as histologic evidence of prolonged inflammation. Other common causes of chronic sialadenitis include radiation, trauma, and immunocompromised conditions.

Signs and symptoms

The symptoms are usually a painful swelling of the gland and pyrexia. They may be associated with meals. Bacterial sialoadenitis is generally unilateral whereas viral sialoadenitis is traditionally bilateral. Pressure over the affected gland may lead to pus leaking from the duct. There may be a palpable stone in the duct or within the gland.

Treatment

Treatment involves rehydration, antibiotics, and attention to oral hygiene. Sialogogues, such as lemon drops that stimulate saliva production, are helpful. Surgical drainage may be required if an abscess complicates this infection.

Chronic salivary gland inflammation or recurrent acute attacks of sialadenitis may arise as a result of stones or stricture within the gland or duct. Stones arise as accumulations of calcium and other salts found in saliva, deposits on foreign material, and food debris within the ducts. Strictures most often occur after an episode of inflammation in the duct. Pain and swelling when eating are common. This condition usually occurs in the submandibular gland, and surgical excision may be required.

Sialolithiasis

Sialolithiasis, or salivary stones, is common and usually affects the submandibular gland, since the secretions are richer in minerals such as calcium and phosphate and thicker because of increased mucin content. The stones are usually composed of hydroxyapatite. About 80%–90% of calculi occur in the submandibular gland, with the remainder occurring in the parotid. There are very few cases of salivary gland stones in the sublingual or minor salivary glands. The stones may cause salivary stasis and obstruction. Risk factors include male gender, prolonged dehydration, gout, diabetes, and hypertension.

Signs and symptoms

Symptoms may include pain and swelling in the affected gland during or after meals. The gland will become tense and tender. Inspection of the floor of the mouth may reveal the thickened, inflamed submandibular duct, and a stone maybe palpable within the duct. If there is any uncertainty about the diagnosis, a plain X-ray or a sialogram (an X-ray of the duct system using dye) should be used. A non-contrast CT scan can also detect stones and defines its relationship to the gland. Submandibular gland stones are generally radio-opaque and visible on radiographs. Most parotid gland stones are radiolucent.

Treatment

Conservative treatment with rehydration, analgesia, and sialogogues may be all that is required. Sometimes a small stone will spontaneously pass out of the duct into the mouth and the symptoms will settle. Larger stones may need to be removed. This can be performed transorally if the stone is palpable in the floor of mouth and near the duct orifice. If the stone is close to the gland, the whole gland may need to be removed by an open operation via the neck. Endoscopic evaluation and removal of calculi have also been described, and lithotripsy for stones has been used.

Other inflammatory conditions

Sjogren syndrome

Sjogren syndrome is an autoimmune disease that afflicts primarily women in their 60's. It causes dry mouth (xerostomia), dry eyes (keratoconjunctivitis sicca), and, in many cases, diffuse, non-tender enlargement of the parotid gland. It may occur in a primary form or be associated with other autoimmune diseases such as rheumatoid arthritis or systemic lupus erythematosus.

There are often circulating antibodies, called autoantibodies SS-A and SS-B, that may be detected in the serum. The diagnosis can be confirmed by biopsy of a minor saliva gland found in the mucosa of the oral cavity, generally the lower lip. Pathology reveals an infiltration of plasma cells around the gland.

Treatment is based on levels of symptoms and is supportive. Systemic steroids may be necessary during acute flares. Steroid eye drops are useful temporarily for severe symptoms. Dry mouth is generally treated with good hydration, artificial saliva, and oral gel. Complications over time include dental caries, difficulty swallowing, and mucosal discomfort. Patients with primary Sjogren syndrome should be followed for the development of lymphoma, which occurs in approximately 10%.

Other causes of salivary gland swelling

Benign lymphoepithelial lesions are associated with HIV infection and are very commonly seen in the parotid gland. Symptoms include a soft, compressible, cystic swelling of the gland which when aspirated yields clear, straw-colored fluid. FNA of the cyst walls may show aciner atrophy and infiltration of lymphocytes with epithelial cells. There is an association with B-cell lymphoma.

Systemic viral infections such as mumps and HIV may cause inflammation of the parotid or submandibular glands.

Necrotizing sialometaplasia is a benign, self-limiting inflammatory process that primarily afflicts males. It appears as a painless ulceration of the hard palate. Histologically, there is squamous metaplasia and pseudoepitheliomatous hyperplasia. The importance of this entity lies in the potential for misdiagnosis as a malignancy such as squamous cell carcinoma or mucoepidermoid carcinoma.

Granulomatous conditions such as tuberculosis and sarcoidosis may affect the saliva glands.

Sarcoidosis is the great mimicker that can present as salivary gland swelling. This systemic granulomatous condition has a wide range of different manifestations and has primarily lung involvement with perihilar lymphadenopathy. Histology shows the presence of non-caseating granulomas. *Heerfordt syndrome* is nonpulmonary sarcoidosis with the following symptoms: parotid swelling, uveitis, facial palsy (secondary to granulomatous inflammation around the facial nerve), sensorineural hearing loss, and fever.

Inflammatory pseudotumor occurs as painless swelling and can affect lymph nodes. This is a non-neoplastic reactive swelling of unknown etiology. Histologically it shows diffuse inflammatory cells with connective tissue. This condition resolves spontaneously.

Pseudosalivary swellings

These swellings may mimic salivary gland enlargement, such as the following:
- Intraglandular lymph nodes
- Hypertrophy of the masseter muscle—may mimic parotid enlargement
- Parapharyngeal space masses—may present as an intraoral mass in a similar way to a deep lobe of parotid mass
- Lesions or cysts of the mandible or teeth—may look like a submandibular gland mass
- Winging of the mandible—may mimic parotid swelling

Salivary gland surgery

See Figs. 7.3–7.5 showing incisions (Fig. 7.3), the facial nerve and its relation to the parotid (Fig. 7.4), and the submandibular gland and anatomy (Fig. 7.5).

The facial nerve passes through the parotid gland and is at risk in parotid surgery. Surgeons will often use the facial nerve monitor to help them identify and avoid injury to the facial nerve.

Other surgical pointers to the position of the facial nerve are listed below:

- The facial nerve exits from the stylomastoid foramen, which lies at the root of tympanomastoid suture. This is palpable during parotid surgery.
- The facial nerve lies approximately 1 cm deep and 1 cm inferior to a small V-shaped piece of cartilage of the tragus known as the tragal pointer.
- The facial nerve bisects the angle made between the mastoid process and the posterior belly of the digastric muscle.
- A retrograde approach may be found by finding a distal branch and tracing the nerve proximally.
- The vertical segment of the facial nerve can be identified via mastoidectomy.

Complications of parotid gland surgery

- Paresthesia or numbness of the ear lobe is common, because the greater auricular nerve may need to be divided to gain access to the parotid gland.
- Hematoma
- Salivary fistula—when saliva leaks out through the incision
- Temporary facial nerve weakness—occurs in about 10% of cases
- Permanent facial nerve weakness—occurs in less than 1% of cases
- Frey's syndrome—sweating and redness of the skin overlying the parotid gland when eating. It occurs when postsynaptic secretomotor nerve fibers are severed during surgery and they re-grow abnormally, innervating the sweat glands of the skin.

Complications of submandibular gland surgery

- Hematoma—the most common complication
- Weakness of the marginal mandibular nerve—this can usually be avoided by making a low, horizontal incision 2 cm below the angle of the mandible. The surgical dissection should be carried out deep to the capsule of the gland, i.e., in a plane deep to the nerve.
- Lingual and hypoglossal nerve damage—these nerves lie close to the deep surface of the gland and are potentially at risk during the surgery.

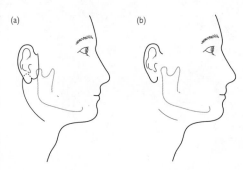

Fig. 7.3 (a) Incision for parotid surgery; (b) incision for submandibular surgery.

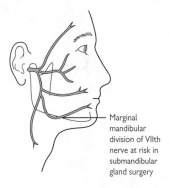

Marginal
mandibular
division of VIIth
nerve at risk in
submandibular
gland surgery

Fig. 7.4 Diagram of facial nerve and it relation to the salivary glands.

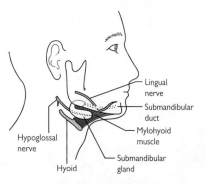

Lingual
nerve

Submandibular
duct

Mylohyoid
muscle

Hypoglossal
nerve

Submandibular
gland

Hyoid

Fig. 7.5 Diagram of submandibular gland and anatomy.

The larynx

Structure and function of the larynx

Structure

The larynx is a tube made up of a cartilaginous skeleton, intrinsic and extrinsic muscles, and a mucosal lining. The cartilaginous skeleton, which houses the vocal cords, is comprised of the thyroid, cricoid, and arytenoid cartilages. Above, the larynx connects with the pharynx and oral cavity; below, it connects with the trachea and major bronchi (Fig. 8.1). Behind the larynx is the opening of the esophagus.

The larynx is suspended from the hyoid bone, which is significant in that it is the only bone in the body that does not articulate with any other bone. The cartilaginous skeleton of the larynx is composed of three unpaired and three paired cartilages. The thyroid cartilage is the largest of the unpaired cartilages and resembles a shield in shape. The second unpaired cartilage is the cricoid cartilage, whose shape is often described as a "signet ring." The third unpaired cartilage is the epiglottis, which is shaped like a leaf.

The three paired cartilages include the arytenoid, cuneiform, and corniculate cartilages. The arytenoids are shaped like pyramids, and because they are a point of attachment for the vocal cords, allow the opening and closing movement of the vocal cords necessary for respiration and voice. The cuneiform and corniculate cartilages are very small and have no clear-cut function. Food and drink are guided from the mouth to the esophagus, while air passes via the trachea to the lungs. Food passes over the back of the tongue and runs down two channels called the piriform fossae. These lie slightly behind and to the side of the larynx. They join behind the cricoid cartilage and form the esophagus (see Fig. 8.2).

Function

The larynx has three primary functions: phonation, respiration, and deglutition. These functions are all intimately related to one another in as much as dysfunction of one affects the other two. For example, during deglutition the larynx protects the lower airways from contamination by fluids, liquids, and saliva. The sequence is as follows: the larynx rises during swallowing, bringing the laryngeal inlet closer to the tongue base and allowing the food bolus to pass on either side. The epiglottis folds down to cover the larynx. The vocal cords and false cords (see Fig. 8.3) come together.

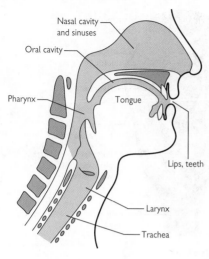

Fig. 8.1 Vocal tract.

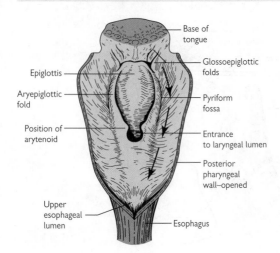

Fig. 8.2 External view of the larynx.

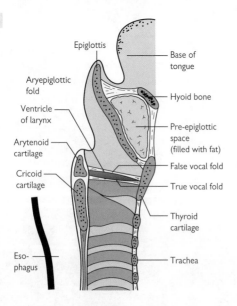

Fig. 8.3 Internal side view of the larynx.

The vocal cords

Structure

The vocal cords, also called the vocal folds, are fixed to the thyroid cartilage at the front and to the arytenoid cartilages at the back. These cartilages can slide away from and toward each other, opening and closing the laryngeal inlet. They divide the larynx in two—the supraglottis lies above the vocal cords while the subglottis lies below.

The mucosal cover of most of the upper airway is respiratory epithelium with numerous mucosal glands. The free edge of the vocal cords is adapted for periodic vibration and is made up of nonkeratinizing squamous mucosa with no mucus glands. A highly specialized lamina propria separates the epithelium from the underlying muscle. This lamina propria contains three layers: superficial, intermediate, and deep. The deep layer is the stiffest layer and is made up of the vocal ligament (part of the conus elasticus). The intermediate layer has the most elastic fibers of the three. The superficial layer is often referred to as Reinke's space and has the lowest concentration of both elastic and collagenous fibers, thus offering the least impedance to vibration.

Innervation

The sensation of the supraglottis and glottis is carried by the internal branch of the superior laryngeal nerve. The external branch carries motor fibers to the cricothyroid muscle. This muscle is important in adjusting the tension of the vocal cord. The vagus nerve gives rise to the recurrent laryngeal nerve and this in turn carries sensation to the subglottis and is motor to all the other muscles of the larynx. The left recurrent laryngeal nerve has an unusually long course and loops down into the chest, lying close to the hilum of the lung. It is prone to infiltration by tumors of this region (see Fig. 8.8, p. 183).

Lymph drainage

The vocal cords are a watershed for lymphatic drainage. Above, the supraglottis drains to the pre-epiglottic and upper deep cervical nodes, while below, drainage is to the lower deep cervical and pretracheal nodes. The cords have very poor lymph drainage, so tumors limited to vocal cords have a low risk of lymphatic spread. Tumors of the lymphatic-rich supra- or subglottis frequently present with lymph node metastases and consequently will have a worse prognosis (see Fig. 8.4, p. 167).

Function

The vocal cords are the source of the sound vibration (phonation), which is further refined with our mouth, tongue, lips, and teeth to produce speech. As air passes up between the cords, the Bernoulli effect draws the mucosa of the cords together. They meet for a fraction of a second and then the pressure rises below the cords, blowing them apart again. This vibration of the cords along with the distortion of the mucosa that results from it is known as the mucosal wave. This is the basis for voice production.

Deglutition is a complex process that relies on several sphincters in the upper digestive tract and is typically divided into three phases. The oral phase is volitional and begins with preparation of the food bolus. As this bolus passes into the vallecula, the involuntary oropharyngeal phase begins. As the food bolus passes through the upper esophageal sphincter the final (esophageal phase) commences.

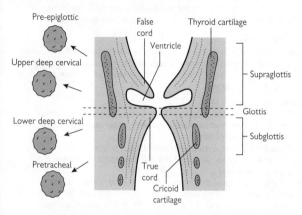

Fig. 8.4 Lymph drainage of the larynx.

Congenital laryngeal lesions

Young children and infants are more prone to breathing difficulties because their larynx differs from that of an adult in the following ways:

- The airway is smaller both relatively and absolutely.
- The laryngeal mucosa is less tightly bound down and as a result may swell dramatically.
- The cartilaginous support for the airway is less rigid than in an adult. This makes it more prone to collapse, especially during inspiration.

Laryngomalacia

Laryngomalacia is the most common cause of stridor in infancy. Furthermore, it is the most common congenital laryngeal anomaly. Males are affected twice as often as females. Laryngomalacia arises from a continued immaturity of the larynx.

Signs and symptoms

- These are often not present at birth. In fact, onset of symptoms typically occurs days to weeks after birth (most commonly within the first 2 weeks of life).
- Typical stridor associated with laryngomalacia is low in pitch, with a fluttering quality secondary to the circumferential rimming of the supraglottic airway and aryepiglottic folds.
- Symptoms are most prominent when the child is in the supine position or when the child is agitated. More forceable inspiration tends to result in a louder stridor quality due to greater prolapse and thus greater obstruction.

Diagnosis

- Radiographic studies can suggest the diagnosis of laryngomalacia, although the mainstay of diagnosis is flexible nasopharyngoscopy.

Treatment

- GERD is associated with and worsens this condition. Patients should be placed on medications to control acid.
- More then 95% of laryngomalcia will resolve in 12–18 months without any interventions.
- Surgical intervention is rare and includes aryepiglottoplasty.

Subglottic stenosis (SGS)

This abnormality can be congenital or acquired. The vast majority (95%) of cases are acquired. The most common cause of acquired SGS (90%) is endotracheal tube intubation. The most important risk factor for the development of laryngotracheal stenosis (LTS) is the duration of intubation. Other factors include size of the endotracheal tube, movement of the endotracheal tube, traumatic intubation, number of re-intubations, and presence of an infection while intubated. Gastro-esophageal reflux (GER) has been proposed as a medical condition that may exacerbate the pathogenesis of LTS, may cause restenosis after repair, and may be the sole cause of stenosis in patients with no previous history of endotracheal intubation or laryngotracheal trauma.

The main sign of this condition is stridor at any age from birth to 2 years. Diagnosis is made by inspecting and measuring the diameter of the subglottis under general anesthetic. The important things to document during endoscopy are as follows:

(1) Outer diameter of the largest bronchoscope or endotracheal tube that can be passed through the stenotic segment
(2) Location or subsites (glottis, subglottis, trachea) and length of stenosis
(3) Other separate sites of stenosis
(4) Other airway anomalies in infants (clefts, webs, cricoarytenoid joint fixation, neoplasms, etc.)
(5) Reflux changes

Mild cases may be treated conservatively, but more severe stenoses require surgical intervention and laryngotracheal reconstruction. See Table 8.1 for grading of stenosis.

Laryngeal web

This condition occurs when the larynx fails to completely recanalize and the airway is reduced. Fusion can be minimal, with little effect on the airway; or complete fusion can occur which is incompatible with life.
The main signs of this condition are respiratory difficulties, stridor, and a hoarse cry. Severe cases will require immediate surgical intervention either via a tracheostomy (when an artificial breathing hole is made in the neck below the cords to bypass the obstruction) or by endoscopic division of the web.

Laryngeal cleft

This occurs when the posterior larynx fails to fuse. At its most severe it will also extend down to involve the posterior wall of the trachea.
The main signs are respiratory problems associated with feeding, as a result of aspiration into the trachea. Mild cases can be difficult to diagnose. When there are symptoms, surgical repair may be needed.

Vocal cord palsy

The recurrent laryngeal nerves are long in children and adults, reaching from the skull base down into the chest and back up again to the larynx. Because of their length, they are prone to damage anywhere along their course. Unilateral palsy will cause a weak, breathy cry and feeding difficulties as a result of aspiration, and bilateral palsy will present as marked stridor.

Table 8.1 Congenital laryngeal lesions: Cotton grading of tracheal stenosis

Grade 1	≤50% obstruction
Grade 2	51%–70% obstruction
Grade 3	71%–99% obstruction
Grade 4	No lumen

Infections of the larynx

Acute laryngitis

Inflammation of the larynx may occur in isolation or as part of a general infective process affecting the whole of the respiratory tract. It is very common, often presenting as a sore throat and loss of voice with a cold.

Signs and symptoms
- Hoarse voice
- Pain on speaking and swallowing
- Malaise
- Slight pyrexia
- Examination of the vocal cords will show them to be reddened and swollen.

Treatment
Most patients with acute laryngitis either self-medicate or are treated in the primary-care setting with supportive therapy such as voice rest, simple analgesia, steam inhalations, and simple cough suppressants.

Voice rest is especially important for any professional voice user. Patients should be advised of this and of the risk of hemorrhage into the vocal cord, which can produce permanent adverse effects on the voice.

Chronic laryngitis

Chronic laryngitis is a common inflammation of the larynx caused by many different factors. It often begins after an upper respiratory tract infection (URTI). Smoking, vocal abuse, chronic lung disease, sinusitis, postnasal drip, reflux, alcohol fumes, and environmental pollutants may all conspire together to maintain the inflammation.

Signs and symptoms
- A hoarse voice
- A tickle in the throat or a feeling of mucus in the throat
- A patient who is constantly clearing their throat or coughing—this causes still more inflammation of the cords and establishes a vicious circle
- A laryngoscopy that reveals thickened, red, edematous vocal cords.

Patients should be referred for a laryngeal examination if their symptoms fail to settle within 4 weeks. If any concern remains after this examination, a biopsy under general anesthetic should be performed to exclude laryngeal malignancy.

Treatment
The agents causing the chronic laryngitis should be removed. The patient may require the skills of a speech therapist. Patients will also respond well to explanation and reassurance that they do not have a more serious condition.

Reinke's edema

This is a specific form of chronic laryngitis found in smokers. The vocal cords become extremely edematous and filled with a thin, jelly-like fluid. The edema fails to resolve because of the poor lymph drainage of the vocal cord. Smoking cessation and speech therapy are helpful in removing the causes of this condition. In some cases microlaryngeal surgery is required to incise the cord and aspirate the edema. It is important to minimize damage to the free edge of the vocal cord when performing this operation, as it can permanently affect the mucosal wave and, hence, the voice.

Epiglottitis and supraglottitis

This is an inflammation of the epiglottis or supraglottic tissues that affects children and adults. Epiglottitis is now uncommon in children (as a result of the HIB vaccination). It is seen more often in adults, where it tends to affect the whole of the supraglottic tissues (and is called supraglottitis).

The causative agent is usually *H. influenzae.*

Signs and symptoms

- Difficulty in swallowing, leading to drooling of saliva
- Change in the voice, described as a muffled or "hot potato" voice, or change in the child's cry
- Dramatic swelling of the supraglottic tissues
- Pools of saliva seen collected around the larynx on endoscopy

This condition should not be underestimated. It may start with features similar to those of any other respiratory tract infection, but it can rapidly progress to total airway obstruction within hours of onset. Consider this diagnosis early on, and get expert help.

Management

- Admit the patient and keep them upright. Laying the patient flat could obstruct their airway.
- Do not attempt to examine the mouth, as this may obstruct the patient's breathing.
- X-rays do not add much to the diagnosis and remove the patient from immediate expert assistance should the patient need it.
- Early diagnosis is essential for reducing morbidity and mortality.
- Call for airway assistance—an otolaryngologist, trauma surgeon, or an anesthesiologist.

Treatment

If epiglottitis or supraglottitis is suspected, stop further investigations. Escort the patient calmly and quickly to an operating room where the anesthesiologist and surgeon are standing by with the appropriate equipment (laryngoscope, ventilating bronchoscope, and tracheostomy set).

Where possible, intubate the patient and treat with the appropriate antibiotics. However, oral intubation may be difficult and surgery may be necessary to secure the airway.

Croup

This infection is common in children. It affects the whole of the upper respiratory tract, hence the more descriptive name, acute laryngo-tracheobronchitis. It is usually viral in origin (parainfluenza most common), but a secondary bacterial infection (staphylococci, pneumococci) is sometimes seen. The speed of onset of croup is slower than in epiglottitis, but it can be extremely serious and even life threatening. Classically, a febrile URTI is followed by a "barky" croupy-like cough. On lateral neck X-rays the classic "steeple" sign is often seen.

Signs and symptoms
- Mild preceeding upper respiratory tract infection
- Rising pyrexia
- Stridor
- Malaise.
- Supraglottis unaffected

Treatment
- Admission to the hospital may be necessary for treatment in a croup tent.
- Intravenous antibiotics (for bacterial superinfection)
- ± racemic epinephrine and nebulizer treatments
- Humidified air and ventilator support if necessary
- Steroids

Cancer of the larynx

The vast majority of laryngeal cancers are squamous cell carcinomas. Smoking is the risk factor for laryngeal cancer, although smoking and drinking in combination puts the patient at even more risk. It is the most common neck and head malignancy.

Since the entire upper aerodigestive tract has been exposed to the same risk factor (i.e., tobacco and alcohol), there is a widespread field change throughout this mucosa. These patients thus have an increased risk of developing another cancer in the mouth, pharynx, larynx, or esophagus. Five percent of patients with one head and neck cancer will present with a second primary tumor elsewhere in the head or neck. This second primary tumor may be entirely asymptomatic.

Signs and symptoms

The patient's symptoms will depend on which site(s) within the larynx is affected. A tumor on the vocal cord will cause a hoarse voice, and a patient in this situation will usually present with symptoms early in the course of disease. However, a tumor in the supraglottis may produce few symptoms until much later and a patient may present with advanced disease. All patients with a mass in the neck must be referred for an ENT examination.

Signs of advanced laryngeal cancer are the following:
• Pain—often referred to the ear
• Voice change—the voice is muffled rather than hoarse, unless the tumor also extends to the true vocal cords.
• Breathing difficulties and stridor
• Difficulty swallowing or inhaling
• Lymph node enlargement in the neck—this is often the only presenting feature.

Investigations

Although a clinical diagnosis can often be made after examination of the larynx, a biopsy is essential, because conditions such as laryngeal papillomas, granulomas, and polyps may mimic laryngeal cancer. All patients should also have an examination of the entire upper aerodigestive tract (panendoscopy) to check for a second primary tumor.

All patients must have at least a chest X-ray. A CT scan of the chest is routine practice in many centers. CT/MRI scanning of the neck is also mandatory, particularly when looking for thyroid cartilage erosion and enlarged lymph nodes in the deep cervical chain.

Staging

TNM staging is applied to head and neck cancers in a similar way to that for other sites.
• The T stage is determined by the anatomical site or sites affected.
• The N stage refers to the local nodal spread.
• The M stage is determined by the presence or absence of distant metastases (see Boxes 8.1–8.3).

Box 8.1 T staging of laryngeal cancer

TX	Tumor cannot be assessed
Tis	Carcinoma in situ
T1a	Tumor limited to one vocal cord
T1b	Tumor involves both vocal cords
T2	Tumor spreading upward or downward from the cord to involve the supraglottis or subglottis and/or impaired vocal cord mobility
T3	Tumor limited to the larynx with vocal cord fixation and/or invades paraglottic space, and/or minor thyroid cartilage erosion (e.g., inner cortex)
T4a	Tumor invades through the thyroid cartilage and/or invades tissues beyond the larynx (e.g., trachea, soft tissues of neck, including deep extrinsic muscle of the tongue, strap muscles, thyroid, or esophagus)
T4b	Tumor invades prevertebral space, encases carotid artery, or invades mediastinal structures

Box 8.2 N staging for the head and neck

N1	A single ipsilateral node, <3 cm in size
N2a	A single ipsilateral node >3 cm but <6 cm in size
N2b	More than one ipsilateral node <6 cm in size
N2c	A contralateral node or bilateral nodes <6 cm in size
N3	Any node >6 cm in size

Box 8.3 M staging for the head and neck

M0	No distant metastases
M1	Distant metastases

Treatment of laryngeal cancer

Premalignant lesions or carcinoma in situ can be treated surgically by removing the entire lesion. Some clinicians advocate the use of a CO_2 laser to accomplish this, but there are concerns about accuracy of review of the pathology. Early-stage laryngeal cancer (T1 and T2) can be treated with either radiation therapy or surgery alone. In this setting they offer about the same 85%–95% cure rate. Surgery has a shorter treatment period, and saves the option of radiation for reoccurrence, but may have worse voice outcomes. The procedure of choice is usually a partial laryngectomy. Radiotherapy is given for 6–7 weeks; its use avoids surgical risks (see Box 8.4, p. 177), but it does have complications, including mucositis, odynophagia, laryngeal edema, xerostomia, esophageal stricture, laryngeal fibrosis, radionecrosis, and hypothyroidism.

Current treatment of advanced laryngeal cancer is evolving. For instance, new chemotherapeutic regimens are undergoing clinical trials. Surgical techniques are changing to decrease the morbidity of total laryngectomy. For advanced-staged lesions, patients usually receive surgery and radiation, most often with surgery before adjuvant radiation. For most T3 and T4 lesions a total laryngectomy is required; some small T3 lesions can be treated with a partial laryngectomy. The adjuvant radiation is started within 6 weeks of the surgery, and with once-daily protocols lasts 6–7 weeks. Indications for postoperative radiation include T4 primary, bone/cartilage invasion, extension into soft tissue of the neck, perineural invasion, vascular invasion, multiple positive nodes, nodal extracapsular extension, margins less than 5 mm, positive margins, carcinoma in situ at margins, and subglottic extension of primary tumor.

Induction and concurrent chemotherapy with external-beam radiation is increasingly being used for the treatment of advanced-stage laryngeal cancer.

Each patient should be assessed individually, and treatment decisions must be made in a multidisciplinary team setting, with the knowledge and consent of the patient.

Surgery for laryngeal cancer

The decision of which type of surgery to perform depends largely on the size and extent of the tumor. Surgery may be performed endoluminally—with endoscopes from the inside—usually with the aid of a laser. Or the radical excision of part of or the entire larynx may be needed. In general, smaller tumors (T1 and T2) are more easily treated with endoscopic laser surgery, and larger T3 and T4 tumors are treated with radical excisional surgery (see Laryngectomy, p. 177).

Box 8.4 Key learning points in radiotherapy for laryngeal cancer

- Treatment intent maybe palliative or curative.
- Chemotherapy is only used as an addition to radiotherapy (or surgical) treatment.
- Small tumors do very well.
- Radiotherapy is usually given for small tumors.
- Large tumors are usually treated with a laryngectomy.
- Postoperative radiotherapy is often given for advanced disease with poor histology.

Laryngectomy

Several different types of partial laryngectomy have been described. These are collectively known as "less than total" and are beyond the scope of this book.

A *total laryngectomy*, first described at the beginning of the last century, remains a reliable and effective treatment. During a total laryngectomy the larynx is removed and the trachea is brought to the skin as an end stoma in the neck. The pharynx is opened and repaired to reconstitute the swallowing mechanism (see Fig. 8.5). A neck dissection is often performed in combination with this procedure because patients with advanced or recurrent laryngeal disease are at considerable risk of having nodal metastases, which may be palpable or hidden.

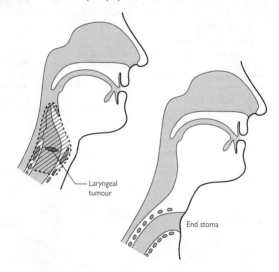

Laryngeal tumour

End stoma

Fig. 8.5 Diagram of pre- and post-laryngectomy anatomy.

Voice restoration after laryngectomy (see also p. 177)

Esophageal speech

In those who can achieve it, esophageal speech (see Fig. 8.6a) offers near-normal verbal communication. The basic principle is that air is swallowed into the stomach and then regurgitated into the pharynx. This causes vibration of the pharyngoesophageal (PE) segment, similar to in a belch. This can be modified with the lips and teeth into intelligible speech.

The main problem is that not all patients can manage to achieve this type of speech, and even if they do, only small amounts of air can be swallowed. This means that the resultant speech can only be made up of short phrases at best.

Tracheoesophageal puncture

In this procedure (see Fig. 8.6b), artificial communication is created between the back wall of the trachea and the front wall of the pharynx/esophagus. This is usually done at the time of the initial surgery (primary puncture), but it can be performed any time thereafter (secondary puncture).

A one-way valve is inserted into this tract, which allows the passage of air from the trachea to the esophagus, vibrating the PE segment as above. To activate the valve, the patient must occlude their stoma and try to breathe out. This may be done with a finger or by using a second manually operated valve that sits over the stoma as part of a heat and moisture exchanger (HME). The HME also filters the inhaled air and prevents excess water vapor from being lost from the respiratory tract—in effect, this replaces some of the functions of the nose.

Artificial larynx (Servox)

Some patients cannot achieve either of the above forms of speech and require an external vibrating source. The vibrating end of this device is held firmly onto the patient's neck, floor of their mouth, or cheek, causing these tissues to vibrate. As a result, the air within the pharynx and oral cavity vibrates and sound is produced. Although the voice produced does sound rather unnatural, this is a simple and effective means of communication (see Fig. 8.7).

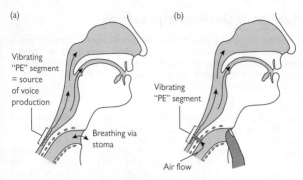

Fig. 8.6 (a) Diagram of esophageal speech and (b) tracheoesophageal puncture.

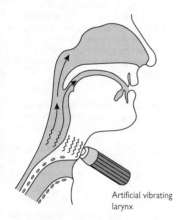

Fig. 8.7 Diagram of Servox.

Benign lesions of the larynx

These are laryngeal lesions that are not cancer. Signs of a benign lesion, such as a hoarseness, can be indistinguishable from those of laryngeal cancer. It is therefore imperative that any patient with a change in their voice lasting more that 4 weeks be referred to an ENT surgeon to exclude a laryngeal malignancy.

Vocal cord polyps

Vocal fold polyps are benign lesions of the middle membranous vocal fold that arise as a result of vocal hemorrhage. They arise spontaneously and suddenly and may be associated with previous laryngeal inflammation. The point at the anterior third of the membranous vocal fold represents the area of pronounced phonotrauma. This region is also known as the "striking zone," and is a region where polyps, nodules, varices, and sulcus commonly form. The symptoms are usually a sudden onset of hoarseness with vocal strain and sore throat.

The appearance of vocal cord polyps can vary widely. Polyps are unilateral and are commonly associated with a reactive fibrous lesion on the contralateral vocal cord. They can be hemorrhagic with evidence of recent hematoma formation. They can be also be pedunculated and may be difficult to see because they sometimes hang down on their stalk to sit below the cords. Histologically, these lesions form within the subepithelial basement membrane. Treatment is with microphonosurgery.

Vocal cord cysts

These lesions are mucus-filled masses within the vocal fold. They usually arise spontaneously and their exact etiology is unknown. They may be associated with previous laryngeal inflammation. The symptoms are a hoarse voice and/or a sore throat.

The cysts are intracordal and can be within the lamina propria or the vocalis muscle. Treatment is with microsurgical excision, taking care to avoid iatrogenic damage to the free edge of the vocal cord and, hence, the mucosal wave and voice.

Vocal cord granuloma

This lesion is usually unilateral and affects the posterior aspect of the vocal cord. As a result, it can have quite a minimal effect on the voice. Vocal cord granuloma arises as a result of inflammation of the arytenoid cartilage (perichondritis). It is most often seen as a result of intubation trauma or excessive coughing. The patient usually complains of pain in the larynx. Reflux is a commonly associated feature.

The lesion may require a biopsy, as SCC can present with similar features. Treatment may include surgical excision, speech therapy, and treatment of acid reflux.

Vocal fold varices and ectasias

Varices and ectasias of the vocal folds are the result of microvascular trauma within the superficial lamina propria. Most of these lesions are located on the superior aspect of the middle membranous vocal fold (striking zone). This condition is most prevalent in vocal abusers, specifically female singers. Voice therapy is the primary modality of treatment. Surgical intervention may be instituted in patients who cannot accept residual vocal symptoms and limitations. One of the more commonly used techniques involves making use of epithelial cordotomies and removing the vessels.

Singer's nodules

These nodules, also known as screamers' nodules, occur as a result of prolonged voice abuse or misuse. They are common in children and amateur actors and singers—they give a characteristic huskiness and strain to the voice.

These nodules are always bilateral and occur at the junction of the anterior third and posterior two-thirds of the vocal cords. Early or "soft" nodules will resolve with speech therapy and good vocal habits, but long-established "hard" nodules may require surgery.

Papillomas

These noncancerous growths are most commonly seen in children but may also occur in adults. Papillomas arise as a result of human papilloma virus (HPV). The route of transmission is thought to be through inhalation. There may also be some defect in the host immune system, as some individuals are affected and others are not. Spontaneuous resolution tends to occur in children around puberty, but this is less common in adults.

In its most severe form, papilloma may result in significant airway obstruction in the larynx, trachea, and major bronchi. If the patient's airway is obstructed, surgical debulking of the papilloma is required. Removal of every last papilloma in not advised, since this will cause scarring of the vocal cords and the papillomas often recur. A tracheostomy should be avoided to prevent spread to the lower airway.

Malignant transformation may occur in adults, especially with subtypes 7 and 11. Systemic treatment with interferon is effective, but rebound growth may be dramatic when it is stopped. Cidofovir and indole 3 carbinol have been used with some success.

Muscle tension dysphonia

This is a common problem seen in general practice and ENT practice. The symptom is a hoarse voice that tires easily and may vary in pitch. Patients sometimes say their voice "cracks" or "gives out" and the quality of the voice varies from day to day and moment to moment. Occasionally the patient may present with aphonia.

These problems are caused by laryngeal muscular-tension abnormalities and are associated with voice misuse, psychological stress, and psychiatric disease.

Globus-type symptoms are frequent, including a feeling of a lump in the throat, a feeling of mucus in the throat, and frequent throat clearing. The treatment is reassurance and explanation, with speech therapy for patients who do not respond well.

Vocal cord palsy

Palsy or paralysis of the vocal cords will mean that the patient may have a weak, breathy voice rather than the harsh, hoarse voice of laryngeal cancer. Patients will have a poor, ineffective cough and aspiration is common. See Box 8.5, p. 183.

The recurrent laryngeal nerve (RLN) is a branch of the vagus nerve and has a long course (see Fig. 8.8, p. 183). This makes it susceptible to damage in a variety of sites (see Fig. 8.9, p. 184).

Investigation

Remember the rule of thirds below:

- 1/3 idiopathic
- 1/3 surgery
- 1/3 neoplasia

Where there is no history of recent surgery, consider the following:

- CT scan—skull base to aortic arch
- Ultrasound of thyroid
- Esophagoscopy

If these images are negative, then postviral neuropathy is the most likely cause. The causes of vocal cord immobility (fixation rather than palsy) include rheumatoid arthritis, laryngeal trauma, prolonged intubation, and carcinoma affecting the cricoarytenoid joint. An endoscopy, together with palpation of the joint, is necessary to confirm this abnormality.

Treatment

Where there is a small gap between the cords, speech therapy may be all that is needed to strengthen the mobile cord and aid compensation. When there is a larger gap, the paralyzed cord can be medialized, either by an injection technique or via thyroplasty (see Fig. 8.10, and Fig. 8.11, p. 184). Poor function of the cords may lead to aspiration and pulmonary infections. Dietary modifications, tube feeding, and even a tracheostomy may be required to protect the airway from aspiration.

Neurological laryngeal conditions

Spasmodic dysphonia (or laryngeal dystonia) is a voice disorder caused by involuntary movements of one or more muscles of the larynx or voice box. Spasmodic dysphonia causes the voice to break or to have a tight, strained or strangled quality. There are three different types of spasmodic dysphonia:

Adductor spasmodic dysphonia is the most common of these conditions and is characterized by abnormal breaks when the vocal cords inappropriately close causing choppy or strained speech. **Abductor spasmodic dysphonia** is characterized by inappropriate opening of the vocal cords and breathy breaks on connected speech. The third type is **mixed** and has features of both.

Currently the best treatment for reducing the symptoms of spasmodic dysphonia is injections of very small amounts of botulinum toxin directly into the affected muscles of the larynx. The injections generally improve the voice for a period of 3–4 months, after which the voice symptoms gradually return. Re-injections are necessary to maintain a good speaking voice. Initial side effects that usually subside after a few days to a few weeks may include a temporary weak, breathy voice or occasional swallowing difficulties.

Box 8.5 Learning points—vocal cord palsy (see Fig. 8.9, p. 184)

- Unilateral vocal cord palsy leads to vocal cord lateralization and a weak voice but a good airway. Over time, the paralyzed cord can medialize or the contralateral cord overcompensates to produce a good voice.
- Bilateral vocal cord palsy leads to vocal cord medialization and airway problems but a good voice.

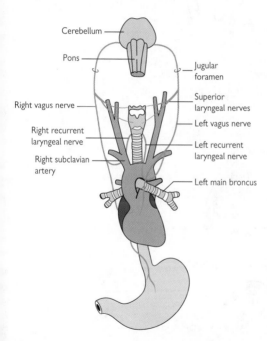

Fig. 8.8 Diagram of recurrent laryngeal nerve anatomy and sites of damage.

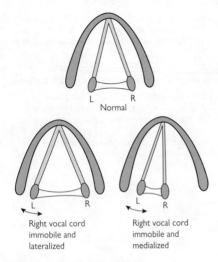

Fig. 8.9 Diagram of palsy positions.

Normal

Right vocal cord
immobile and
lateralized

Right vocal cord
immobile and
medialized

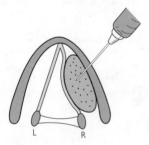

Fig. 8.10 Diagram of injection.

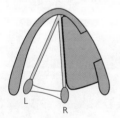

Fig. 8.11 Diagram of thyroplasty.

Stridor

Stridor is usually a high-pitched noise caused by an obstructed airway. It is most common in children, because of the anatomical differences between the pediatric and the adult larynx (see p. 162).

The timing of the stridor in respiration tells you the site of the obstruction or restriction:

- Laryngeal stridor = inspiratory
- Tracheal stridor = expiratory—a wheeze
- Subglottic stridor = biphasic—occurs when breathing in or out

A small reduction in the diameter of the airway leads to a dramatic increase in airway resistance and, hence, the work of breathing (Poiseuilles law: resistance $= r^4$).

Causes of stridor

Congenital

- Laryngomalacia
- Vocal cord web
- Bilateral vocal cord palsy
- Subglottic stenosis

Acquired

- Trauma
- Foreign body
- Epiglottitis or supraglottitis
- Croup
- Carcinoma
- Airway compression, e.g., thyroid

Assessment

Stridor is an ominous sign. Even if the patient appears to be coping, be sure that they are closely observed and that facilities to secure the airway are readily at hand. Patients may suddenly decompensate with devastating consequences.

- Take a rapid history.
- Measure O_2 saturation.
- Take the patient's temperature.
- Check respiratory rate.

In children, pyrexia, drooling, dysphagia, and a rapid progression of the illness suggest epiglottitis. Take the patient to a place of safety such as a resuscitation room or operating room and call for a senior ENT surgeon and experienced anesthetist.

A similar history in adults suggests supraglottitis. This diagnosis can usually be confirmed by careful nasolaryngoscopy.

Also see the section on emergency airway, below.

The emergency airway

Remember to keep calm!

The following questions should be answered first:

- Will admission and observation be sufficient for the time being, or do you need to intervene to secure the airway?
- If intervention is required, do you need to do something now, or do you have time to wait for help to arrive?

Assessment

Assessment should follow three stages: look, listen, and observe.

Look

- What is the patient's color—is he or she blue?
- Are there any intercostal retractions or tracheal tug?
- What is the patient's respiratory rate?

Listen

- Can the patient talk in sentences, phrases, words, or not at all?
- Do they have stridor? Is it inspiratory, expiratory, or mixed?
- What history can the patient give?

Observation

- Is the patient's respiratory rate climbing?
- Is the patient feverish?
- What is the patient's O_2 saturation? Is it falling?

Interventions

Consider the following options:

- Give the patient oxygen via a face mask or nasal prongs.
- Broad-spectrum antibiotics, such as Augmentin (check that the patient is not allergic)
- Racemic ephinephrine
- Systemic steroids
- Heliox—this is a mixture of helium and oxygen that is less dense than air. It is easier to breathe, and it buys you time, during which you can take steps to stabilize the airway.

Endotracheal intubation

This should be the first line of intervention where possible. If it proves difficult or impossible, move on quickly.

Cricothyroidotomy

Any hollow tube can be inserted through the cricothyroid membrane into the airway (see Fig. 8.12). The Bic pen is famous for having been used in this way, but a wide-bore cannula, "mini-trac," or transtracheal ventilation needle is probably more appropriate. If you are unsure of your landmarks, fill a syringe with a little saline and use a needle to probe for the airway, with suction applied. A steady stream of bubbles will appear when the airway is entered.

Tracheostomy

A surgical hole is made in the trachea below the cords. In an emergency, a longitudinal incision is made in the midline of the neck and deepened to the trachea, dividing the thyroid. Brisk bleeding is to be expected. The blade is plunged into the airway and twisted sideways to hold the tracheal fenestration open. A cuffed tracheostomy or endotracheal (ET) tube is inserted into the airway and the bleeding thyroid is dealt with afterwards.

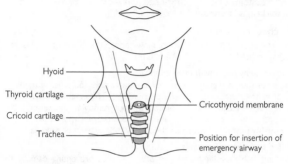

Hyoid

Thyroid cartilage

Cricoid cartilage

Trachea

Cricothyroid membrane

Position for insertion of emergency airway

Fig. 8.12 Cricothyroidotomy.

Tracheostomy care and tracheostomy tubes

Tracheostomy operation

In an elective tracheostomy, the incision is usually placed horizontally. The strap muscles are separated in the midline, and the thyroid isthmus is carefully divided and oversewn. The trachea is opened at the third or fourth tracheal ring, and a window of tracheal cartilage is removed. A tracheostomy tube of the right size (three-quarters of the diameter of the trachea) is inserted and the cuff is inflated.

Tracheostomy tubes

The choice of tubes may seem bewildering; the basic principles are described below (see Figs. 8.13 and 8.14).

Tracheostomy tubes with inner cannula

The inner tube is slightly longer than the outer one, and crusting tends to occur at the distal end and on the inner tube. The inner tube can easily be removed, cleaned, and replaced without removing the outer tube. Any patient who is likely to require a tracheostomy for more than 1 week is probably best fitted with a tracheostomy tube with inner cannula.

Cuffed and non-cuffed tubes

The cuff is high volume and low pressure, thus preventing damage to the tracheal wall. The cuff prevents fluid and saliva from leaking around the tube and into the lungs. In addition, it makes an airtight seal between the tube and the trachea, thus allowing positive-pressure ventilation. Most tubes are cuffed, but when a tracheostomy is in place long term, and no mechanical ventilation is needed, a cuffless tube should be used to prevent damage to the trachea.

Metal tubes

Metal tubes are non-cuffed and are used only for patients with permanent tracheostomies. They have the advantage of being inert and "speaking valves" can be inserted.

Fenestrated tubes

Most tubes are non-fenestrated. The advantage of a fenestrated tube (one with a hole in its side wall) is that air can pass through the fenestration, through the vocal cords and enable the patient to talk. The disadvantage is that they may have an increased incidence of granulation tissue and subglottic stenosis.

Post-tracheostomy care

In the first few days after a tracheostomy operation, special care needs to be taken. The patient should be nursed by staff familiar with tracheostomy care. The patient should be given a pad and pencil with which to communicate.

Precautions
- The tube should be secured with tape and knotted at the side of the neck until a tract is well established.
- The tape should be tied with the neck slightly flexed.
- The cuff should not be overinflated, to prevent ischemic damage to the tracheal wall. Use a pressure gauge to check the cuff's pressure.
- The patient must be given humidification for at least the first 48 hours to reduce tracheal crusting.
- Regular suctioning of the airway to clear secretions may be needed.
- A spare tracheostomy tube and an introducer should be kept by the patient's bed in case of accidental displacement of the tube.
- Tracheal dilators should also be close by for the same reason.

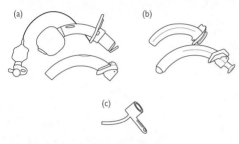

Fig. 8.13 Diagram of tracheostomy tubes. (a) Cuffed fenestrated tube; (b) non-cuffed non-fenestrated tube; (c) pediatric tube.

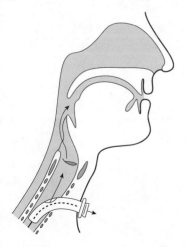

Fig. 8.14 Diagram of tracheostomy tube position (note fenestration).

The esophagus

Introduction

The esophagus is a muscular tube connecting the pharynx to the stomach. In adults it is 25 cm long. It starts at the level of C6, the cricoid cartilage, and it ends at the gastroesophageal junction, or the diaphragm. The cricopharyngeus muscle acts as an upper esophageal sphincter.

Congenital esophageal conditions

These rare conditions may account for some cases of infant death, feeding problems, or failure to thrive. They are frequently associated with other abnormalities of the larynx and/or the trachea. Complex surgery may be required and treatment should be given in specialist pediatric centers (see Fig. 9.1).

Esophageal foreign bodies

See Chapter 20 p. 424, ENT emergencies.

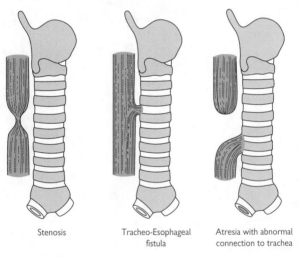

Stenosis   Tracheo-Esophageal   Atresia with abnormal
                         fistula   connection to trachea

Fig. 9.1 Congenital esophageal lesions.

Globus

Globus pharyngeus, syndrome, and hystericus are all terms that have been used to describe a common symptom complex of a "feeling of a sensation in the throat (FOSIT) with no obvious cause." It is probably caused by excess muscle tension in the pharyngeal musculature.

Features

- Feeling of a lump in the throat
- Mucus collection in the throat that is rarely cleared
- Symptoms come and go.
- Symptoms are usually in the midline.
- The sensation is most noted when swallowing saliva rather than food or drink.
- Worse when stressed
- Worse when tired
- More common in women
- Associated with gastroesophageal reflux disease (GERD)

Pharyngeal malignancy may present with similar symptoms, so beware especially of the following

- Unilateral globus
- Globus and otalgia
- Globus and a neck lump
- Persistent or progressive symptoms

Reassurance is usually all that is required to treat globus, but further studies such as barium swallow or endoscopy may be required to exclude malignant disease.

Laryngopharyngeal reflux

Laryngopharyngeal reflux (LPR) is a common condition associated with gastroesophageal reflux (GERD). It is caused by changes in the larynx and upper aerodigestive tract due to stomach acid reflux. It is often associated with an incompetent lower esophageal sphincter or hiatus hernia.

Doctors and patients may not recognize that GERD, a stomach problem, could be responsible for their throat symptoms.

Classical symptoms of GERD

- Heartburn
- Discomfort behind the sternum
- Nausea
- Waterbrash—bitter fluid regurgitation
- Odynophagia—discomfort with hot or cold drinks

Laryngopharyngeal reflux symptoms

- Mucus in the throat
- Postnasal drip
- A feeling of a lump in the throat
- Hoarse voice
- Sore throat on waking
- Cough
- Globus

Investigations

Patients with a history of reflux symptoms such as indigestion, heartburn, and burping may be treated with a therapeutic trial of a proton pump inhibitor (PPI) for 1 month.

If the symptoms recur or treatment fails completely, patients should be referred for further investigation with an upper gastrointestinal (GI) endoscopy, barium swallow, and 24-hour pH monitoring.

Conservative treatment

Patients should be advised on the following:
- Make dietary changes such as avoiding spicy food, carbonated drinks, and alcohol.
- Avoid using common triggers that include caffeine, chocolates, and peppermints.
- Try to lose weight if obesity is a problem.
- Avoid going to bed within 3 hours of eating.
- Stop smoking.
- Prop up the head of the bed on a couple of bricks or blocks or use a sleeping wedge.

Medical treatment

- Antacids such as Gaviscon
- H$_2$ antagonists such as ranitidine
- Proton pump inhibitors

Surgical treatment

Patients who are resistant to treatment may require anti-reflux surgery, which can be performed laparoscopically.

Neurological causes of swallowing problems

The mechanics of the upper aerodigestive tract are complex. Food, drink, and saliva are directed toward the esophagus, via the pyriform sinus, while air passes to the lower respiratory tract via the larynx.

The swallowing mechanism is a complex process involving both sensory and motor functions. It is initiated voluntarily but progresses as a dynamic reflex. A neurological condition that affects a patient's motor or sensory function may also cause problems with swallowing.

Common neurological causes of swallowing problems

- CVA (stroke)
- Bulbar palsy
- Motor neuron disease
- Multiple sclerosis
- Tumors of the brainstem
- Cranial nerve lesions, e.g., vagal neuroma
- Systemic neurological conditions, e.g., myasthenia gravis

Investigations

Assessment will involve taking a detailed swallowing history and asking the patient about any coughing or choking attacks indicating aspiration.

A general neurological examination and a specific cranial nerve examination should be done. A chest X-ray may show evidence of aspiration. A video swallow gives detailed information about the function of the esophagus (such as delay, pooling, poor coordination, spasm, cricopharyngeal hyperfunction, etc.). A barium swallow test may be of limited value because it will only give static pictures.

Treatment

Wherever possible, the patient's underlying condition should be treated, but there will be times when the aims of treatment are to control the symptoms. This could involve the following:

- Swallowing therapy as directed by a speech and language therapist
- Dietary modification, such as more thickened fluids
- Gastrostomy feeding tube.
- Cricopharyngeal myotomy—surgical division of the upper esophageal sphincter muscle
- Vocal cord medialization procedures, when a vocal cord paralysis causes aspiration
- Tracheostomy (see p. 187)
- Tracheal diversion or total laryngectomy (see p. 177)

Post-cricoid web

This is a rare condition and its cause is unknown. An anterior web forms in the lumen at the junction of the pharynx and esophagus, behind the cricoid cartilage.

Patterson Brown–Kelly (UK) and Plumber–Vinson (USA) both describe this condition—their names are frequently used in association with the syndrome.

A post-cricoid web is linked with iron deficiency anemia, and it has the potential to become malignant. Because of this chance of malignancy, an endoscopy and biopsy are recommended. It may also cause dysphagia, and can be seen on a barium swallow.

The web may be dilated and/or disrupted with the help of an endoscope.

Achalasia

The specific cause of achalasia is unknown. Patients with achalasia have two problems of the esophagus. The first is that the lower two-thirds of the esophagus does not propel food toward the stomach properly. The second problem is dysfunction of the lower esophageal sphincter (LES). The LES should relax in response to swallowing to allow food to enter the stomach. In patients with achalasia, the LES fails to relax, creating a barrier that prevents food and liquids from passing into the stomach. One theory about achalasia is that the nerve cells responsible for relaxation are destroyed by an unknown cause.

Signs and symptoms
- Progressive dysphagia
- Regurgitation
- Weight loss

Investigations
A barium swallow may suggest achalasia. An endoscopy is needed to exclude an esophageal tumor, as this can produce similar X-ray appearance and symptoms.

Treatment
Drug therapy Two classes of drugs, calcium channel blockers and nitrates. Usually taken 30 minutes prior to meals, they cause relaxation of the sphincter.

Balloon dilatation (pneumatic dilatation) Balloon dilatation mechanically stretches the contracted LES. This procedure is effective for relieving symptoms of achalasia in two-thirds of patients, although chest pain persists in some people. Up to half of patients may require more than one treatment for adequate relief.

Surgery (myotomy) Myotomy can be used to directly cut the muscle fibers of the LES. The surgical technique used most often is called the Heller myotomy. In the past, surgery was performed through an open incision in the chest or abdomen, but it can now be performed through a tiny incision using a thin, lighted tube (a laparoscope or a thoracoscope). This new approach is less traumatic and shortens recovery time. Patients who undergo myotomy are given general anesthesia and generally stay in the hospital for 1–2 nights.

Botulinum toxin injection Botulinum toxin injection is a new treatment for achalasia. The botulinum toxin temporarily paralyzes the LES, preventing contraction and helping to relieve the obstruction. Botulinum toxin injection may also be used as a diagnostic test in people with suspected achalasia who have inconclusive test results.

Zenker's diverticulum

This is a type of hernia, or pulsion diverticulum, that affects the junction of the pharynx and esophagus. Elderly males are most often affected.

Zenker's diverticulum is believed to arise as a result of incoordination of the swallowing mechanism, leading to an increased intraluminal pressure above the closed upper esophageal sphincter. As a result of this pressure, the pharyngeal mucosa herniates through an anatomical area of weakness, known as Killian's dehiscence, that lies between the two heads of the inferior constrictor muscle (see Fig. 9.2).

Signs and symptoms
- Dysphagia
- Regurgitation of undigested food
- Halitosis
- Gurgling noises in the neck
- A lump in the neck
- Aspiration
- Pneumonia

Investigations
A barium swallow will indicate the diagnosis. A rigid endoscopy must follow to exclude the rare finding of a carcinoma within the pouch. This is sometimes the result of long-term stasis of its contents.

Treatment
Treatment is only necessary if the patient is symptomatic. Endoscopic stapling of the wall that divides the pouch from the esophagus is the current treatment of choice. Excision, inversion, and suspension of the pouch have been described.

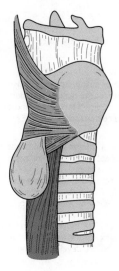

Fig. 9.2 Pharyngeal pouch.

Esophageal tumors

Benign esophageal tumors are rare and arise from the local tissue elements, e.g., leiomyoma, adenoma, lipoma.

Malignant esophageal tumors

The risk factors for a malignant esophageal tumor include smoking, a high alcohol intake, achalasia, and anemia. Eighty percent of malignant tumors occur in males over 60 years old. Primary carcinomas are the most common. These carcinomas are squamous and adenocarcinoma.

Squamous cell carcinoma

Squamous cell carcinoma arises from this epithelial layer in an apparent response to chronic toxic irritation. Alcohol, tobacco, and certain nitrogen compounds have been identified as carcinogenic irritants.

Certain medical conditions predispose patients to the development of esophageal squamous cell carcinoma. These include achalasia, lye strictures, head and neck tumors, celiac disease, Plummer–Vinson syndrome, tylosis, and prior exposure to radiation. Squamous cell carcinoma may arise in the setting of achalasia, typically after a period of 20 or more years, and it is believed to result from long-standing irritation by retained material. Of patients with strictures caused by lye ingestion, 3% develop squamous carcinomas after 20–40 years.

Adenocarcinoma

Most common in the mid- and distal esophagus, adenocarcinoma arises from abnormal esophageal mucosa in a well-characterized sequence. In reaction to chronic gastroesophageal reflux, metaplasia of the normal stratified squamous epithelium of the distal esophagus occurs, resulting in a specialized intestinal glandular epithelium containing goblet cells, called Barrett epithelium. Further genetic alterations in this epithelium lead to dysplasia, which may progress from low-grade to high-grade dysplasia and, ultimately, to adenocarcinoma. Gastroesophageal reflux disease is the most important factor in the development of Barrett epithelium. Of patients with GERD, 10% develop Barrett epithelium. Of patients with Barrett epithelium, 1% develop esophageal adenocarcinoma, a risk that is 30–40 times higher than in the population without Barrett epithelium. Therefore, patients with Barrett epithelium are advised to undergo periodic surveillance esophageal endoscopy with biopsy.

The signs and symptoms

- Weight loss
- Pain in the throat and/or epigastrium
- Progressive dysphagia

Investigations

- Barium swallow may show a narrowing or mucosal abnormality suggesting a malignant tumor.
- Endoscopy and biopsy will confirm the diagnosis.
- CT scan of the chest and abdomen is used to assess the extramucosal extent and metastatic spread.

Treatment

- The best chance of a cure is with surgical excision, where possible. This may be given with preoperative chemotherapy and postoperative radiotherapy.
- After the excision, the resulting esophageal defect will be reconstructed, with either a stomach pull-up, free jejunal grafting, or a myocutaneous flap (see Fig. 9.3).

Where a cure is not possible, palliation may be achieved via
- Radiotherapy
- Laser debulking of the mass
- Endoscopic stenting
- PEG tube for long-term feeding

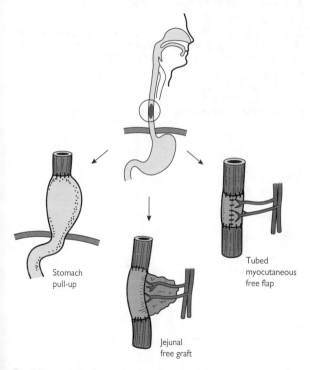

Stomach
pull-up

Jejunal
free graft

Tubed
myocutaneous
free flap

Fig. 9.3 Reconstruction.

Barrett's esophagus

Barrett's esophagus (BE) is a metaplastic disorder in which specialized columnar epithelium replaces healthy squamous epithelium. Barrett metaplasia is the most common cause or precursor of esophageal carcinoma. The rate of esophageal adenocarcinoma is increasing in the Western world, and it has a poor prognosis, mainly because individuals present with late-stage disease. The exact causes of Barrett's esophagus are not known, but it is thought to be caused in part by the same factors that cause GERD. Although people who do not have heartburn can have Barrett's esophagus, it is found about three to five times more often in people with this condition. Barrett's esophagus is uncommon in children. The average age at diagnosis is 60, but it is usually difficult to determine when the problem started. It is about twice as common in men as in women.

Diagnosis

Barrett's esophagus can only be diagnosed by an upper GI endoscopy to obtain biopsies of the esophagus. At present, it cannot be diagnosed on the basis of symptoms, physical exam, or blood tests.

Treatment

- Behavior and diet changes
- Medications—PPI
- Surgery if reflux is uncontrolled by medications

The neck

Anatomy of the neck

Surface anatomy

Many of the important structures in the neck can be seen or felt on examination. These are:
- The mastoid process (a)
- The clavicular heads (b)
- The sternocleidomastoid muscle (c)
- Trachea (d)
- Cricoid cartilage (e)
- Cricothyroid membrane (f)
- Thyroid prominence (g)
- Hyoid bone (h)
- Carotid bifurcation (i)
- Thyroid gland (j)
- Parotid gland (k)
- Submandibular gland (l)
- Jugulodigastric lymph node (m)

Use Fig. 10.1 to identify the above structures on yourself. It is particularly important to quickly identify the cricothyroid membrane to be able to perform an emergency cricothyroidotomy (see p. 205).

Triangles of the neck

The anterior and posterior triangles of the neck are often referred to in clinical practice and are useful descriptive terms. These triangles may be subdivided as shown in Fig. 10.2a, but the usefulness of the subdivisions is questionable.

Deep anatomy

The neck is divided into anatomical compartments by strong fascial layers (see Fig. 10.2b).
- **The posterior compartment** contains the skeletal muscles of the cervical spine.
- **The anterior compartment** contains additional fascial envelopes that have these important structures:
  - The pretracheal fascia encloses the thyroid gland and binds it to the trachea.
  - The carotid sheath encloses the carotid, internal jugular, and vagus nerve.

Between these fascial planes lie the parapharyngeal space and the retropharyngeal space. These spaces are clinically relevant because they may become involved in and allow the spread of deep-seated infections or malignancy.

(a)

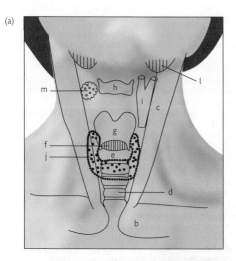

(b)

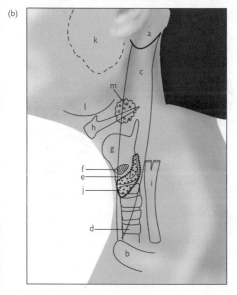

Fig. 10.1 Surface anatomy of the neck.

Lymph node levels

The classification of lymph node levels in the neck is commonly referred to in clinical practice, and it is important to have an understanding of them (see Fig. 10.3).

Most lymph drainage from the aerodigestive tract is through the deep cervical chain, which runs along the internal jugular vein deep to the sternocleidomastoid muscle. It has been discovered that particular anatomical sites drain reliably to particular groups of lymph nodes.

A nodal-level system has been devised to simplify the discussion of lymph nodes and to ensure that we are all talking the same language. Essentially, this is a naming system that gives a number or level to groups of lymph nodes in a particular area. See Fig. 10.3, which is a diagram of the lymph node levels in the neck.

This nodal-level system is of particular importance when considering the lymphatic spread of head and neck cancers. The first group of nodes that a cancer involves is called the first-echelon nodal level. For example, the first-echelon nodes for tonsil cancer are level 3; from here other nodal levels may be affected, usually levels 2 and 4.

Cancers in other sites may metastasize in different patterns, for example, the first-echelon nodes from nasopharyngeal cancer tend to be level 5. This concept and model have led to the development of selective neck dissections, i.e., supraomohyoid neck dissections (see p. 217).

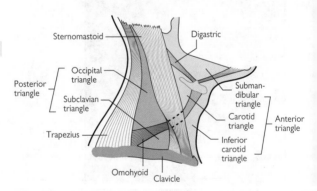

Fig. 10.2a Triangles of the neck.

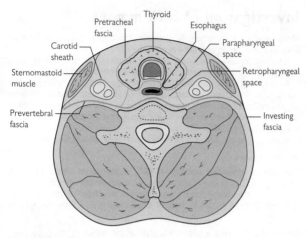

Fig. 10.2b Fascial layers and spaces of the neck.

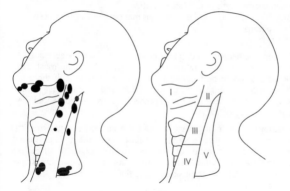

Fig. 10.3 Lymph node levels in the neck.

Investigation of neck masses

Neck masses are common. All patients with a neck mass must have an ENT examination to exclude a malignancy.

A full history should be taken, including duration, change in size, smoking history, pain (including referred otalgia), and any concurrent illness.

A neck mass should be thoroughly examined and the following aspects noted: site, size, shape, texture (smooth or lobulated), position (midline or central), solid or cystic, single or multiple, tender, attached to deep structures, movement on swallowing, movement on tongue protrusion, pulsatile (see Fig. 2.14, p. 33).

In addition to the above, a full ENT examination should be given.

Investigations

Fine needle aspiration cytology (FNAC) is the single most important diagnostic test. It is like a blood test but involves taking cells from the mass rather than blood from a vein. There is no danger of seeding malignant cells if the appropriate method is used (see p. 227, How to perform an FNA).

Blood tests Where the history suggests an inflammatory mass, consider the following:
- Complete blood count (CBC)
- Sedimentation rate or C-reactive protein
- Paul–Bunnell, monospot, or infectious mononucleosis (IM) screen
- Toxoplasma
- HIV test

Biopsy may be needed if a diagnosis cannot be made. Wherever possible, this should be excisional rather than incisional. All but the most trivial neck masses should be biopsied under general anesthesia. If there is a high suspicion of malignancy based on history and clinical finding, frozen sections should be sent and the patient should also be consented for a possible neck dissection.

Endoscopy Cancers of the silent sites of the head and neck may give little or no symptoms themselves but may metastasize to the neck, presenting as a neck mass. Examination of these sites is vital, usually under general anesthetic, i.e., via panendoscopy, which looks at the entire upper aerodigestive tract. The silent sites include the following:
- Nasopharynx
- Tongue base
- Tonsil
- Vallecula
- Pyriform fossa
- Post-cricoid region

Radiology
- Chest X-ray—for malignancy, TB, HIV.
- Ultrasound scan (USS)—for thyroid, salivary glands. This test may be useful in children, as it is noninvasive and easy, and it can distinguish between a solid or a cystic mass.
- Spiral CT—rapid acquisition is useful for mobile structures like the larynx and for those patients who find lying flat difficult.
- MRI—provides excellent soft tissue definition but is degraded by patient movement.

Congenital neck remnants

Thyroglossal cysts and fistulae

The thyroid gland develops at the base of the tongue and descends through the tissues of the neck to its final position overlying the trachea. It leaves a tract that runs from the foramen cecum of the tongue to the thyroid gland. This tract curves around the body of the hyoid bone. Thyroglossal cysts and fistulae arise from congenital abnormalities of this process. They are the most common mass found in the midline of the neck. The mass is usually located at or below the level of the hyoid bone, although a thyroglossal duct cyst (TGDC) can be located anywhere from the foramen cecum to the level of the thyroid gland. They are common in teenagers and in young adults.

Signs and symptoms

These may present as a midline swelling, a paramedian swelling, or a discharging sinus. The cyst will rise on tongue protrusion because of their attachment to the tongue base (see Figs. 10.4, and 11.1, p. 221).

Treatment

Before surgical excision of the lesion, ensure that there is a normal functioning thyroid gland in its usual position in the neck. Surgical excision, known as Sistrunks operation, involves removing the lesion plus the tissue block between the lesion and the hyoid, plus the mid-portion of the hyoid bone and any associated tract passing to the foramen cecum of the tongue. Very rarely, carcinoma can appear in the thyroglossal duct. It is typically papillary adenocarcinoma.

Branchial system

The word *branchial* comes from the Greek "bragchia," meaning gills. A *cyst* refers to a mucosa- or epithelium-lined structure with no external or visceral openings. A *sinus* refers to a tract with or without a cyst that communicates to either the gut or skin. A *fistula* is a tract connecting the gut to the skin. There are several types of branchial cysts or sinuses, depending on their embryological origin.

Types
First branchial cleft cyst

First branchial cleft cysts are divided into type I and type II. Type I cysts are located near the external auditory canal. Most commonly, they are inferior and posterior to the tragus, but they may also be in the parotid gland or at the angle of the mandible. They may be difficult to distinguish from a solid parotid mass on clinical examination. Type II cysts are associated with the submandibular gland or found in the anterior triangle of the neck.

Second branchial cleft cyst

The second branchial cleft accounts for 95% of branchial anomalies. Most frequently, these cysts are identified along the anterior border of the upper third of the sternocleidomastoid muscle, adjacent to the muscle. However, these cysts may present anywhere along the course of a second branchial fistula, which proceeds from the skin of the lateral neck, between the internal and external carotid arteries, and into the palatine tonsil. Therefore, second branchial cleft cyst is in the differential diagnosis of a parapharyngeal mass.

Third branchial cleft cyst

Third branchial cleft cysts are rare. A third branchial fistula extends from the same skin location as a second branchial fistula (recall that the clefts merge during development); however, a third branchial fistula courses posterior to the carotid arteries and pierces the thyrohyoid membrane to enter the larynx. Third branchial cleft cysts occur anywhere along that course (e.g., inside the larynx), but are characteristically located deep to the sternocleidomastoid muscle.

Fourth branchial cleft cyst

Fourth branchial cleft cysts are extremely rare. A fourth branchial fistula arises from the lateral neck and parallels the course of the recurrent laryngeal nerve (around the aorta on the left and around the subclavian artery on the right), terminating in the pyriform sinus. Therefore, fourth branchial cleft cysts arise in various locations, including the mediastinum.

Complications

These include squamous cell carcinoma arising in a branchial cleft cyst.

Treatment

Treatment is with surgical excision. These lesions do not regress and frequently become infected.

Dermoid cysts

These cysts lie anywhere between the chin and the suprasternal notch. They arise from defects in fusion of the midline and are an example of "inclusion cysts." They present as painless midline swellings and do not move on swallowing or tongue protrusion (as in thyroglossal duct cysts). Treatment is via surgical excision.

Hemangioma

A hemangioma is an abnormal proliferation of blood vessels that may occur in any vascularized tissue. Hemangiomas are usually not present at birth but are antedated by a pale, well-circumscribed flat area that may contain some central telangiectasia. The actual hemangioma will appear within the first month and will continue to increase in size for the next 3–8 months. A stable phase of relatively no growth then occurs over the next 6–12 months, followed by slow involution of the tumor by ages 5–7 years. They can occur just about anywhere in the head and neck, but are more common in the skin, parotid, lip, oral cavity, perinasal region, and larynx or subglottis. The complications of these lesions are ulceration, infection, bleeding, compression syndromes (airway compromise), thrombocytopenia, and even high-output cardiac failure.

Various modalities of therapy are used to treat hemangiomas. They depend on a variety of factors including: the age of the patient, the site and size of the lesion, and the hemodynamic flow of the hemangioma. It is important to note that congenital lesions typically regress.

Treatment
- Observation
- Steroids
- Embolization, cryotherapy, sclerotherapy, antifibrinolytic agents
- Radiation therapy
- Laser photocoagulation
- Surgery with or without preoperative embolization
- Any combination of the above

Cystic hygroma

These are rare, benign lymphangiomas found in neonates and infants. They insinuate themselves between the tissues of the neck and may reach a massive size. They may cause compressive airway symptoms.

Treatment involves securing the airway where necessary, surgical excision, which can be staged, or injection with sclerosant.

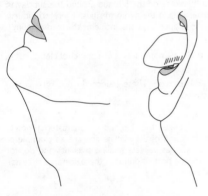

Fig. 10.4 Thyroglossal cysts rise on tongue protrusion.

Neck infections

Parapharyngeal abscess

This is a deep-seated infection of the parapharyngeal space (see p. 207). It often results from a primary infection in the tonsil or is an extension from a parapharyngeal abscess (or quinsy) (see p. 98). It is more common in children than in adults.

Signs and symptoms

These include pyrexia, neck swelling deep to the sternocleidomastoid muscle, and a patient who seems unwell. There may be trismus or a reduced range of neck movements. The tonsil and the lateral pharyngeal wall may be pushed medially. Airway compromise is a late and ominous sign.

If the diagnosis is in doubt, a CT scan will often distinguish between lymphadenitis and an abscess.

Treatment

This will involve a high dose of IV broad-spectrum antibiotics (Unasyn), in addition to surgical drainage.

Retropharyngeal abscess

This is an infection of the retropharyngeal space. It is much more common in children and infants than in adults.

Signs and symptoms

These include an unwell patient with pyrexia, often with preceding URTI or swallowing difficulty. There may be shortness of breath or stridor, or torticollis, due to prevertebral muscle irritation.

Treatment

A high dose of IV broad-spectrum antibiotics (Unasyn) can be given. Where necessary, the airway should be secured, and surgical incision and drainage may be performed via the mouth.

Ludwig's angina

This is a rare infection of the submandibular space; it usually occurs as a result of dental infection. It is more common in adults than in children.

Signs and symptoms

These include pyrexia, drooling, trismus, and airway compromise due to backward displacement of the tongue. There may be firm thickening of the tissues of the floor of mouth, which is best appreciated on bimanual palpation.

Treatment

High doses of IV broad-spectrum antibiotics (Unasyn) can be given. Secure the airway (try a nasopharyngeal airway first, since this will often suffice, but where necessary consider a tracheostomy). Surgical incision is often unsatisfying since little pus may drain away.

Lymph node enlargement

- The majority of neck nodes in children are benign.
- The majority of neck nodes in adults are malignant.
- Neck nodes may be involved secondarily in an infection of any part of the ENT systems.

See p. 206, Lymph nodes.

Nonneoplastic lymphadenopathy
Cervical
- Viral upper respiratory infection
- Infectious mononucleosis
- Rubella
- Cat scratch disease
- Streptococcal pharyngitis
- Acute bacterial lymphadenitis
- Toxoplasmosis
- Tuberculosis or atypical mycobacterial infection
- Acute leukemia
- Lymphoma
- Neuroblastoma
- Rhabdomyosarcoma
- Kawasaki disease

Submaxillary and submental
- Oral and dental infections
- Acute lymphadenitis

Occipital
- Pediculosis capitis
- Tinea capitis
- Secondary to local skin infection
- Rubella
- Roseola

Preauricular
- Local skin infection
- Chronic ophthalmic infection
- Cat scratch disease

The diagnosis in these cases will often be made following the appropriate screening blood test and chest X-ray. FNAC and even excision biopsy may be needed to exclude malignancy.

Neoplastic lymphadenopathy

Lymphoma

This is a primary malignant tumor of the lymphatic tissues.

Signs and symptoms

These include multiple nodes of a rubbery consistency. The patient may or may not experience night sweats, weight loss, axillary or groin nodes, and lethargy.

Investigations

FNAC may produce suspicious findings; an excision biopsy is often required to confirm the diagnosis and allow for subtyping. A chest X-ray and/or a chest CT scan may be done, or, for staging, a CT scan of the abdomen or pelvis. Bone marrow may be needed for staging.

Treatment

This may involve chemotherapy and/or radiotherapy. The patient may need a lymphoma multidisciplinary team review.

Squamous cell carcinoma

This is a primary mucocutaneous malignancy that commonly spreads to local lymph nodes. It can affect single or multiple nodes.

Signs and symptoms

The patient may have ENT-related symptoms such as a sore throat, a hoarse voice, or otalgia. The nodes may have a firm or hard consistency. The patient may have a history of smoking.

Investigations

These may include FNAC, an ENT examination to look for head and neck primary carcinoma, a CT or MRI scan of the neck, a CT scan of the chest and/or chest X-ray (to look for metastases), a whole body PET scan, a liver USS (metastases), a panendoscopy, and biopsy.

Where no ENT primary is seen on examination, a rigorous search should be done for a silent tumor. This will usually involve imaging as above with ipsilateral tonsillectomy, biopsy of the tongue base, postnasal space, and pyriform fossa at a minimum (see Silent areas of ENT, p. 208).

Treatment

This depends on the stage, the size, and the site of the primary tumor (see also Box 10.1). Options for treatment include the following:

- **Radiotherapy** involves 4–6 weeks of daily treatment with a total dose of 50–60 Gy.
- **Radical neck dissection** involves removing the affected nodes as well as all the other nodal groups and lymph-bearing structures on that side of the neck. This includes the lymph nodes at levels 1, 2, 3, 4, and 5, the internal jugular vein (IJV), the sternomastoid muscle, and the spinal accessory nerve.

- *Modified radical neck dissection* takes all the nodal levels (1, 2, 3, 4, 5) but preserves one or all of the IJV, the sternomastoid, and the accessory nerve.
- *Selective neck dissection* Instead of all the nodal groups being removed, those groups thought to be at most risk are selectively dissected and removed. All other structures are preserved.

Box 10.1 N staging of the neck

N1   A single node <3 cm
N2a A single node >3 cm but <6 cm
N2b >1 ipsilateral node <6 cm
N2c Bilateral or contralateral nodes <6 cm
N3   Any node >6 cm

Neck hernias

Pharyngeal pouch
See p. 198.

Laryngocele

This is caused by expansion of the saccule of the larynx. The *saccule* is a blind-ending sac arising from the anterior end of the laryngeal ventricle (p. 164, Fig. 8.2). A *laryngocele* is an air-filled herniation of this structure. This can expand, and either remains within the laryngeal framework (internal laryngocele), or part of it may extend outside the larynx (external laryngocele). It escapes through a point of weakness in the thyrohyoid membrane.

There is a rare association with a laryngeal cancer of the saccule, and all patients should have this area examined and biopsied.

There is little evidence to support the supposition that this condition is more frequent in trumpet players and glass blowers.

Signs and symptoms
- Mass in the neck, which may vary in size
- Hoarseness
- A feeling of something in the throat (FOSIT)
- Swallowing difficulties
- Airway problems

If the laryngocele become infected and full of pus (laryngo-pyocele) then they may rapidly increase in size and cause additional pain.

The thyroid and parathyroid glands

Embryology and anatomy of the thyroid

Thyroid problems are frequent topics in both undergraduate and postgraduate exams. It is thus well worth investing some time in understanding the thyroid.

Embryology of the thyroid

The thyroid begins its development at the foramen cecum at the base of the tongue. The foramen cecum lies at the junction of the anterior two-thirds and the posterior third of the tongue in the midline (see Fig. 11.1).

The thyroid descends through the tissues of the neck and comes to rest overlying the trachea. This descent leaves a tract behind it—this can be the source of pathology in later life (see Box 11.1) (e.g., thyroglossal cysts—see Chapter 10, p. 212).

Anatomy of the thyroid

The thyroid gland is surrounded by pretracheal fascia and is bound tightly to the trachea and to the larynx. This means the gland moves upward during swallowing. The recurrent laryngeal nerves (branches of the vagus) lie very close to the posterior aspect of the thyroid lobes. These nerves have ascended from the mediastinum in the tracheoesophageal grooves and are at risk in thyroid operations. They may become involved in thyroid malignancy; in cases of malignancy a patient will often present with a weak and breathy hoarse voice.

The thyroid gland has a very rich blood supply—trauma or surgery to the gland can lead to impressive hemorrhage into the neck.

The parathyroid glands, important in calcium metabolism, lie embedded on the posterior aspect of the thyroid lobes.

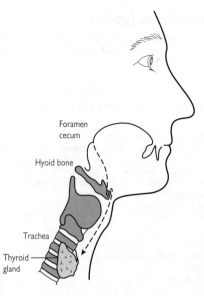

Fig. 11.1 Embryology of the thyroid gland.

Box 11.1 Key points—thyroid-related swellings

- Thyroid masses move on swallowing.
- Thyroglossal cysts move on tongue protrusion (see p. 210).

Thyroid enlargement (goiter)

Goiter simply means an enlargement of the thyroid gland. It is not in itself a diagnosis. Both physiological and pathological conditions may cause a goiter.

Simple goiter

This is a diffuse enlargement of the thyroid and may result from iodine deficiency. Diffuse enlargement of the gland also occurs in Graves' disease.

Multinodular goiter

This benign goiter is the most common thyroid problem. It is caused by episodic periods of thyroid hypofunction and subsequent thyroid-stimulating hormone (TSH) hypersecretion, which leads to hyperplasia of the gland. This is followed by involution of the gland. Prolonged periods of hyperplasia and involution are thought to be responsible for the nodular enlargement of the gland found in a multinodular goiter.

A finding of a single nodular enlargement of the thyroid raises the question of malignancy. This should be managed as described below (see Fig. 11.2).

Treatment

A partial thyroidectomy may be necessary, but only in a patient with one or all of the following signs:

- Pressure symptoms in the neck
- Dysphagia
- Airway compression
- Cosmetic deformity

Graves' disease

This disease is an autoimmune condition in which antibodies are produced that mimic the effect of TSH. A hyperthyroid state develops and there is often a smooth goiter. There is an associated hypertrophy of the orbital muscles causing exophthalmos. The Graves' ophthalmopathy may be most impressive (the actor Marty Feldman had this condition). See p. 226 for eye signs in Graves' disease.

Treatment

Treatment is hormonal manipulation with carbimazole. Surgery to correct the proptosis may be achieved via a transnasal orbital decompression. Here, the medial wall of the bony orbit is removed to allow the orbital contents to herniate into the nasal cavity.

Hashimoto's thyroiditis

This is an autoimmune condition characterized by the destruction of thyroid cells by various cell- and antibody-mediated immune processes. There can be a transient hyperthyroidism, but most patients present with hypothyroidism. Many patients develop a goiter, but the gland can be normal sized or atrophic. Hypothyroidism is usually insidious in onset, with signs and symptoms slowly progressing over months to years. Thyroxine replacements may be necessary. Patients with this condition have an increased risk of developing a thyroid lymphoma.

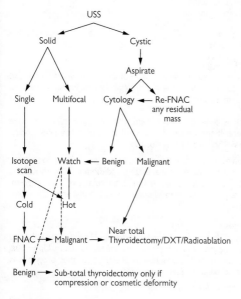

Fig. 11.2 Management of a thyroid lump.

Thyroid neoplasia

Thyroid tumors may arise from either the follicular cells or the supporting cells found in the normal gland. They are quite common, and each of these tumors has its own particular characteristics (see Fig. 11.3). Papillary and follicular adenocarcinomas are frequently referred to as differentiated thyroid tumors.

Follicular cell neoplasms

- Papillary adenocarcinoma
- Follicular adenocarcinoma
- Anaplastic adenocarcinoma

Supporting cell neoplasms

- Medullary carcinoma

Papillary adenocarcinoma

This adenocarcinoma usually affects adults of age 40–50 years. There are usually multiple tumors within the gland. Papillary carcinoma spreads via the lymphatic system, hence 60% of presenting patients have involved neck nodes.

If the disease is limited to the gland, 90% of patients will survive 10 years or more. If the disease has spread to involve the neck nodes, 60% of patients will survive 10 years or more.

Treatment involves a total thyroidectomy, plus a neck dissection where there are involved nodes. A postoperative radioiodine scan should be performed and if increased uptake is found, an ablative dose is given. After surgery, patients will need lifelong thyroid replacement at TSH-suppressing doses.

Follicular adenocarcinoma

This type usually affects adults of age 50–60 years. There is a well-defined capsule enclosing the tumor, and it spreads via the bloodstream. Up to 30% of patients will have distant metastases at presentation, thus prognosis is poorer than that for papillary adenocarcinoma.

Treatment is as above for papillary adenocarcinoma.

Anaplastic thyroid carcinoma

This condition occurs in adults over 70 years of age, and is more common in women. It involves rapid enlargement of the thyroid gland and pain. The patient will have airway, voice, or swallowing problems due to direct involvement of the trachea, larynx, or esophagus.

The prognosis is very poor, with 92% of patients with this condition dying within 1 year, even with treatment.

Medullary carcinoma

This carcinoma arises from the parafollicular C cells (or calcitonin-secreting cells). The patient's level of serum calcitonin is raised and their serum calcium level remains normal. Neck metastases are present in up to 30% of patients.

Treatment involves a total thyroidectomy and radiotherapy.

Benign thyroid adenoma

These adenomas can be functioning or nonfunctioning.

Functioning adenomas

These adenomas produce thyroxine and will take up iodine and technetium. They appear bright, or "hot," on isotope scanning. Symptoms of thyrotoxicosis may develop. They are rarely malignant.

Although treatment is usually medical with thyroid-suppressing drugs, it may be surgical via excision. Radiotherapy and ablation may be required.

Nonfunctioning adenomas

These adenomas do not take up iodine. They appear "cold" on isotope scanning, with 10%–20% being malignant. Treatment is via surgical excision.

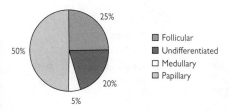

Fig. 11.3 Distribution of thyroid tumors.

Thyroid investigations

Before performing any special investigations, look for signs of abnormal thyroid function. Classic signs are given Table 11.1.

Table 11.1 Classic signs of abnormal thyroid function

Hyperthyroidism	Hypothyroidism
Irritability	Mental slowness
Heat intolerance	Cold intolerance
Insomnia	Hypersomnolence
Sweatiness	Dry skin
Amenorrhea	Menorrhagia
Weight loss	Weight gain
Diarrhea	Constipation
Palpitations	Bradycardia
Hyperreflexia	Slow-relaxing reflexes
Tremor	Loss of outer third of eyebrow
Atrial fibrillation	Hoarse voice

Graves' disease gives rise to particular eye signs:
- Lid lag
- Exophthalmos
- Ophthalmoplegia
- Lid retraction
- Proptosis
- Chemosis

Blood tests

Thyroid function tests (TFTs)

T4 (thyroxine) and T3 (tri-iodo-thyronine) are both bound to plasma proteins in the blood, but a proportion of both remains unbound and is physiologically active. Bear this in mind when interpreting these results in conditions where the free-to-bound ratio may be disturbed, e.g., in nephrotic syndrome or pregnancy.

Thyroid-stimulating hormone (TSH) controls the production of thyroid hormones via a negative feedback mechanism. TSH is usually raised in hypothyroidism and reduced in hyperthyroidism.

Thyroglobulin

This is the carrier protein for T4. Its levels can be measured directly in the blood. It is most frequently used as a tumor marker for the differentiated thyroid carcinomas.

Calcitonin

This is produced by the medullary C cells of the thyroid. Levels are raised in medullary thyroid carcinomas.

Carcinoembryonic antigen (CEA)

This is a tumor marker of medullary carcinoma of the thyroid.

Thyroid autoantibodies

Specific thyroid autoantibodies can be identified in Graves' disease and Hashimoto's thyroiditis.

Radioisotope scanning

Radiolabeled iodine (^{123}I) or technetium (^{99}Tc) is given to the patient orally. Then radiology is used to assess its subsequent uptake into metabolically active thyroid tissue. A thyroid nodule may take up the marker—it will appear bright, or "hot," or it will fail to accumulate the marker and it will appear "cold."

- 80% of thyroid nodules are "cold."
- 10%–20% of "cold" nodules are malignant.
- "Hot" nodules are usually benign.
- Often does not obviate the need for fine needle aspiration cytology

Ultrasound scan (USS)

This is an excellent investigation for demonstrating the thyroid. It will readily distinguish solid and cystic masses inside the thyroid. Often, a USS will show that what appears clinically as a single nodule is in fact part of a multinodular goiter.

MRI and CT scans

CT and MRI are not a routine component of the thyroid mass evaluation. The use of iodine as intravenous contrast for CT scans will interfere with radioactive iodine therapy and should be avoided if a well differentiated thyroid malignancy is suspected.

These scans may be helpful in determining the extent of a retrosternal swelling. A non-contrast CT scan of the neck and chest may confirm airway distortion or compression from a large goiter. These scans may also reveal nodal metastases.

Fine needle aspiration cytology (FNAC)

This test can be used to differentiate solid from cystic masses and it may help in diagnosing malignancy. A residual mass noted after cyst aspiration should be tested again by FNA to exclude malignancy. Papillary carcinoma is diagnosed by the presence of nuclear grooves and intranuclear inclusions (often described as "Orphan Annie eyes"). It is difficult to distinguish between follicular adenoma and follicular carcinoma; the difference lies in demonstrating capsular invasion, which is impossible to show on cytological features alone. Formal histology is usually required to confirm this diagnosis.

Treatment of thyroid conditions

Management of a thyroid nodule

This is best shown diagrammatically; see the flow chart in Fig. 11.2, p. 223.

Hormonal manipulation

Thyroxine Patients experiencing hypothyroid states and those who have undergone thyroidectomy may need to take thyroxine for life. Doses of thyroxine sufficient to suppress TSH production are given in well-differentiated thyroid cancers to reduce tumor growth, since these tumors are also TSH driven.

Carbimazole or propylthirouracil may be given in hyperthyroidism, since these inhibit the formation of T3 and T4.

Radioactive ablation

Most well-differentiated thyroid tumors will trap iodine. This ability can be put to therapeutic effect by administering radioactive iodine. The patient is first rendered hypothyroid via thyroidectomy. The tumor cells then become hungry for iodine and will avidly take up the radioactive iodine to their own cytotoxic demise! Radioiodine therapy can also be used to control a persistent hyperthyroid state.

Thyroid surgery

Thyroid surgery is generally safe and well tolerated by patients.

Hemithyroidectomy involves the removal of one thyroid lobe. It is indicated in benign thyroid conditions and as an excisional biopsy procedure when malignancy is suspected but not confirmed.

Total thyroidectomy is indicated in thyroid malignancy. Because it increases the risks to the recurrent laryngeal nerves and to the parathyroid glands, some surgeons will perform a near-total thyroidectomy, leaving a small amount of thyroid tissue behind in the area of the recurrent laryngeal nerve.

Risks and complications of thyroid surgery

Discussed below are some of the most common and important risks of thyroid surgery.

Vocal cord palsy

This is due to recurrent laryngeal nerve damage. Patients will present with a weak and breathy voice. All patients should undergo a vocal cord check preoperatively to document cord mobility before the procedure.

Bilateral vocal cord palsy

This will lead to medialization of the vocal cords, resulting in life-threatening airway obstruction. Facilities for re-intubation and tracheostomy must be readily available.

Hematoma

Hematoma after thyroid surgery is another potentially serious complication because the vascular nature of the thyroid can lead to a rapid accumulation of blood in the neck, resulting in compression of the airway. For this reason, all thyroidectomy patients should have stitch/clip removers at the bedside. If a patient's neck begins to swell rapidly after thyroid surgery, the wound should be reopened (on the ward if necessary), the clot evacuated, and the airway restored. Once the airway has been secured, the bleeding point can be found and controlled.

Hypocalcemia

This should be anticipated whenever a total thyroidectomy has been performed. Daily calcium levels should be checked and the patient should be observed for the signs of hypocalcemia:

- Tingling in the hands and feet
- Perioral paraesthesia
- Muscle cramps
- Carpopedal spasm—muscle spasms affecting the hands and feet
- Chvosteck's sign—facial spasm seen on tapping over the facial nerve in the region of the parotid
- Tetany—generalized muscle spasm

As soon as hypocalcemia is suspected, give the patient IV calcium gluconate and start oral replacement therapy.

Parathyroid embryology and function

Embryology

In all vertebrate species, the parathyroid glands are derived from the endoderm of the pharyngeal pouches. The superior parathyroid glands are derived from the fourth pharyngeal pouch. During development, they are intimately associated with the lateral lobes of the thyroid gland, to which they become anchored, giving them a consistent location (usually midway along the posterior thyroid borders, where the inferior thyroid artery enters the gland or at its intersection with the recurrent laryngeal nerve). The inferior parathyroid glands are derived from the third pharyngeal pouch. During development, they are intimately associated with the thymus gland and have a more inconsistent location than the superior parathyroid glands. They are usually found close to the inferior thyroid poles, but may descend with the thymus into the thorax or may not descend at all, remaining above the carotid bifurcation. Accessory or supernumerary parathyroid glands are found in approximately 13% of individuals at autopsy.

Function

The function of the parathyroid glands is to maintain the body's calcium level within a very narrow range. When blood calcium levels drop below a certain point, calcium-sensing receptors in the parathyroid gland are activated to release parathyroid hormone (PTH, also known as parathormone) into the blood.

PTH is a small protein that takes part in the control of calcium and phosphorus homeostasis, as well as bone physiology. Parathyroid hormone has effects antagonistic to those of calcitonin. It increases blood calcium levels by stimulating osteoclasts to break down bone and release calcium. It also increases gastrointestinal calcium absorption by activating vitamin D, and promotes calcium uptake by the kidneys.

Hyperparathyroidism

There are three classic types of hyperparathyroidism—primary, secondary, and tertiary.

Primary hyperthyroidism

Primary hyperthyroidism accounts for most instances of hyperparathyroidism. Patients usually present with a finding of hypercalcemia with normal renal function. Malignancy must be ruled out in patients with hypercalcemia and an elevated PTH level. Primary hyperparathyroidism is usually the result of a single benign adenoma; a minority of patients will have hyperplasia of all four parathyroid glands. Parathyroid carcinoma accounts for an insignificant minority.

Secondary hyperparathyroidism

Secondary hyperparathyroidism is due to resistance to the actions of PTH, usually from chronic renal failure. The bone disease in secondary parathyroidism along with renal failure is termed renal osteodystrophy.

Tertiary hyperparathyroidism

Tertiary hyperparathyroidism is a rare form caused by long-lasting disorders of the calcium feedback control system. When the hyperparathyroidism cannot be corrected by medication, one calls it tertiary hyperparathyroidism.

Symptoms

Depending on the severity of the hypercalcemia and the duration of the disorder, a variety of symptoms can occur. Most cases of primary hyperparathyroidism are asymptomatic. For late symptoms remember the mnemonic, "painful bones, renal stones, abdominal groans, and psychic moans"!

Treatment

Surgery to remove the enlarged gland (or glands) is the main treatment for the disorder and cures it in 95% of operations.

Familial hypercalciuric hypercalcemia (FHH)

Also known as familial benign hypercalcemia, this is an autosomal dominant disorder caused by a defect in a calcium-sensing receptor gene. This disorder has similar symptoms to those of the more common primary hyperparathyroidism. It is important to differentiate the two because parathyroidectomy is inappropriate in treatment of this disorder. Differentiation from primary hyperparathyroidism can often be achieved by measuring the renal calcium/creatinine clearance ratio, which generally is less than 0.01 in patients with FHH and higher in patients with primary hyperparathyroidism.

The external ear

Structure and function

A working knowledge of the anatomy of the ear helps in documentation and correspondence and in describing sites of lesions and trauma over the telephone. The main anatomical points are shown in Figs. 12.1. and 12.2.

The external part of the ear consists of two parts:
- The pinna
- The external auditory canal (EAC)

The pinna collects sound waves and directs them into the external auditory canal. Its shape helps to localize sound direction and amplification. The EAC helps in transmitting sound waves to the eardrum or tympanic membrane.

The EAC has two parts:
- An outer cartilaginous part
  - In adults, the cartilaginous canal slopes forward and downward.
  - In neonates and infants, the canal slopes forward.
  - The outer canal contains hairs and ceruminous glands that produce wax.
- An inner bony part

(a) (b)

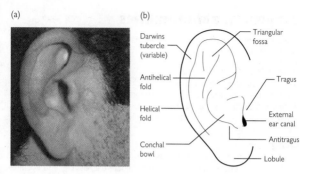

Fig. 12.1 Diagram of the pinna.

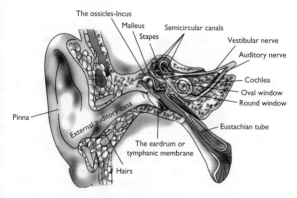

Fig. 12.2 Diagram of the external auditory canal.

Congenital abnormalities

Minor abnormalities of the ear are common, but often they do not come to medical attention.

Malformed pinna

The pinna develops from the six hillocks of His. Maldevelopment or failure to fuse can produce obvious abnormalities of the ear. Malformed pinna are described as microtia or anotia. They may or may not be associated with middle or inner ear abnormalities. The various classifications are shown in Fig. 12.3.

Investigations

This includes documenting the defect, examining the EAC, and doing a hearing assessment. A CT scan to assess middle ear, ossicle, and cochlea anatomy may also be done.

Treatment

- Where there are minor anatomical abnormalities, no treatment is given or hearing support is given as required.
- Where there is a major deformity or anotia, reconstruction of the pinna may be considered. Consider a bone-anchored hearing aid (BAHA) and abutments for attaching an artificial pinna.

Skin tags

Preauricular or periauricular skin tags are often detected at a neonatal baby check. They are often incidental. Investigations involve checking for normal EAC and screening hearing.

Preauricular sinus

This is a small dimple anterior to the tragus. It is usually detected at a baby check and is caused by the incomplete fusion of the hillocks of His. This preauricular dimple may be the external opening of a network of channels under the skin. Patients who present late may have a discharge from the punctum. Occasionally, repeated infections may require drainage.

Treatment

Where there is simple discharge, treat with oral antibiotics such as Augmentin. Where there are repeated infections, antibiotics may be given and surgical removal may be necessary (Fig. 12.4).

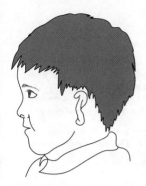

Fig. 12.3 Diagram of microtia grade III. Grading of microtia: I, normal ear; II, all pinna elements present but malformed; III, rudimentary bar only; IV, anotia.

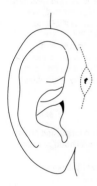

Fig. 12.4 Diagram of preauricular sinus.

Infection of the pinna

This would present as a painful, hot, red ear.

Investigations
- Identify the cause of the infection. Is this a spreading infection from the EAC or is it a primary infection of the pinna?
- Identify whether it is an infection of the skin or whether it involves cartilage. If the cartilage is infected, there is severe tenderness on touching the pinna (see Box 12.1).
- Take a history and exclude trauma or an insect bite. Remember to consider nonaccidental injury in children. Diabetic or immunocompromised patients may have severe cellulitis of the pinna.

Treatment
- Where there is a localized infection, remove any cause such as jewelry piercing or an insect's sting. Give oral antibiotics such as Ciprofloxain or Augmentin.
- Where there is cellulitis of the pinna, remove the cause and treat with IV antibiotics such as cefuroxime 1.5 g 8 hourly and metronidazole 500 mg tid IV 8 hourly until cellulitis resolves, for at least 24 hours, followed by oral antibiotics for 1 week in total.
- Where there is perichondritis, remove the cause and treat otitis externa if present. Treat with Ciprofloxacin or IV antibiotics such as cefuroxime 1.5 g 8 hourly and metronidazole 500 mg tid IV 8 hourly until cellulitis resolves, for at least 24 hours, followed by oral antibiotics for 1 week in total.

Box 12.1 Piercings
- Trends in fashion dictate that piercings are often multiple and not in the lobule of the ear. Lobule piercings have less likelihood of infection, as there is no cartilage in the lobule.
- Other piercings transfix the cartilage framework of the pinna. This can lead to infection and cellulitis of the pinna.

Trauma to the pinna

Assess the patient, bearing in mind that a blow to the ear is a head injury. Discover the force and mechanism of the injury. The site of the injury should be carefully documented with the help of a diagram or a photograph.

Any blunt trauma to the ear may cause a hearing loss or a traumatic perforation of the eardrum. Always examine the EAC drum and perform a simple bedside hearing assessment as follows:

- Examine the pinna and note the findings.
- Examine the EAC.
- Examine the tympanic membrane.
- Perform tuning fork tests.
- Perform free-field testing of hearing.
- Check patient's tetanus status.

Lacerations of the skin

These are simply repaired, using nonabsorbable sutures such as 5.0 Prolene. Apply local anesthetic to the area, clean the wound, and use interrupted sutures. Pay careful attention to everting the edges and ensuring good opposition of the skin edges. Check the patient's tetanus status.

Lacerations involving the cartilage

- Clean wounds can be simply sutured in layers to include the cartilage.
- The cartilage is very painful to suture and a general anesthetic (GA) may be required.
- Dirty wounds may need surgical debridement before closure.
- All wounds require antibiotic cover such as Ciprofloxacin or Augmentin.

Hematoma of the pinna

This is a collection of blood between the perichondrium and the cartilage which leads to pressure necrosis of the cartilage. Subsequent deformity, infection, and fibrosis with cartilage loss lead to the typical "cauliflower ear" of the wrestler.

Aspiration of the hematoma is difficult because of the thickness of the clot. It is better to incise the hematoma and suture, using bolsters to prevent re-accumulation (see Fig. 12.5).

Treatment

- Local anesthetic (LA) or GA
- Incision over hematoma
- Dental roll bolsters tied in place
- Removal of dressing after 5 days
- Oral antibiotics.

(a)

(b)

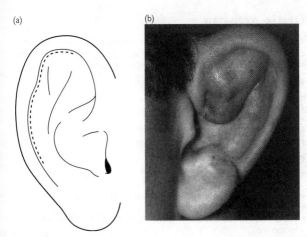

Fig. 12.5 Hematoma of pinna.

Otitis externa

This common condition forms a large percentage of both the emergency and routine workload of an Otolaryngology department. Its presentation is varied and it produces a spectrum of disorders, classified below.

Risk factors

- Swimmers and surfers
- Diabetics
- Immunosuppressed patients (HIV)
- Psoriasis sufferers
- People with an abnormal migration of keratin

Clinical grading

- Is the pinna normal? If there is cellulitis, admission may be needed—severe otitis externa (OE)
- What is the appearance of the EAC after cleaning under microscope?
- Is the EAC of normal diameter?—mild OE
- Is the EAC narrow but the tympanic membrane (TM) still visible?—moderate OE
- Is the EAC narrow but the TM not visible due to edema?—severe OE
- Is there a furuncle in the EAC?
- Are there granulations in the floor of the EAC? This may be necrotizing OE (see p. 244)
- Test the patient's facial nerve function.

Treatment

All patients should keep ears water-free during treatment.

Mild OE

Presentation is scaly skin with some erythema. Treat as follows:

- Use either 0.5% hydrocortisone cream prn to be applied to the EAC,
- Acetic acid ear drops. Lowering of the pH changes the flora of the EAC.
- Perform regular aural toilet and avoid swimming.

Moderate OE

Presentation is of painful, discharging, smelly ears. There is a narrowed EAC with cream cheese–like discharge. Treat as follows:

- Do microsuction clearance.
- Swab for microscopy if there has been previous antibiotic treatment.
- Otowick if the EAC very narrow.
- Use hygroscopic drops, e.g., aluminium acetate.
- Change wick in 48 hours.
- Swab if no improvement. Consider combination therapy with antibiotic steroid drops depending on swab result and response to treatment.

Severe OE

Presentation is complete occlusion of the EAC or spreading pinna cellulitis. Treat as follows:

- Do microsuction clearance.
- Treat as moderate OE.
- If there is severe pain, it may be furunculosis. Lance boil with a needle or fine end of sucker. Add Ciprofloxin 500 mg bid po to regime.
- If there is cellulitis, admission for IV antibiotics may be needed.
- Exclude the tympanic membrane during treatment.

Be aware of allergy

Patients not responding to the appropriate therapy may be allergic to the constituents of the drops. Patch testing may help to elucidate this problem.

Necrotizing otitis externa

This is an uncommon, severe, bacterial ear infection where the infection spreads beyond the ear canal and into the surrounding bone. It is also known as malignant otitis externa because of the mortality associated with the condition. It is usually seen in diabetics or immunocompromised patients. If you see a diabetic patient with otitis externa, consider this condition.

Signs and symptoms
- Otalgia is out of proportion to the clinical appearance of the EAC.
- There is granulation tissue in the floor of the EAC at the junction of the bony and cartilaginous parts of the canal.
- Microvascular disease predisposes to an osteomyelitis that spreads across the skull base. Cranial nerves VII and IX–XII may be affected. The opposite side of the skull base can be affected.
- *Pseudomonas* is the most common pathogen on culture.

Management
- Admit patient for assessment.
- Take a full history.
- Make a thorough ENT examination.
- Check cranial nerves.
- Perform an aural toilet.
- Perform a biopsy of the ear canal under GA or LA to exclude malignancy
- Do a CT scan to examine the appearance of the skull base and to stage the extent of the disease.
- Give ciprofloxacin drops.
- Give oral ciprofloxacin.
- Involve the infectious disease team.
- Continue with drug therapy for 6–12 weeks.
- Perform a surgical debridement only if the patient does not respond to treatment or if there is skull base extension.

Be aware of malignancy
If things fail to settle or if the condition progresses, don't forget, there may be a possible malignant cause. An initial negative biopsy may be wrong. Consider further deep biopsy or cortical mastoidectomy for histology.

Malignancy of the pinna

- The pinna is a common site for malignant skin lesions to develop.
- The types of cancer are basal cell carcinoma (BCC), squamous cell carcinoma (SCC), and malignant melanoma.

Risk factors

- Sun exposure
- Previous skin cancers
- Chemical exposure
- Xeroderma pigmentosum.

Investigations and treatment

It is sometimes possible to make a diagnosis based on clinical observation. Usually excision biopsy is the treatment of choice. Histological examination can confirm the type of malignancy. Further wider excision with or without grafting can be undertaken.

Special reconstructions of the pinna

The unique appearance and structure of the pinna lead to several methods of reconstruction after tumor removal. The aim is to preserve the structure of the pinna and its cosmetic appearance without compromising curative removal. See Fig. 12.6.

If there is gross cartilage involvement, it may be necessary to remove the pinna entirely.

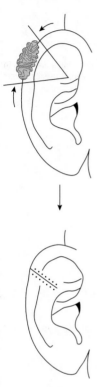

Fig. 12.6 Diagram of wedge resection.

Malignancy of the external auditory canal

This is a rare condition, but it forms an important differential diagnosis in dealing with infections or masses in the ear. When seen, it usually affects the elderly. SCC is the most common type of malignancy.

Signs and symptoms
- A growth in the EAC
- An otitis externa
- Facial nerve palsy
- Other cranial nerve palsies such as IX–XII
- Lymph node metastases

Management
- Treat any infection.
- Biopsy the lesion.
- Perform CT scan to stage the lesion.
- Perform MRI scan to assess intracranial spread.

Treatment options
- Palliative
- Curative
- Radiotherapy
- Surgery

Prognosis
The outlook for these patients is universally poor, with low 5-year survival rates.

Miscellaneous conditions

Exostoses

Exostoses are the most common bony abnormality of the EAC; they are present in approximately 1 out of every 150 patients examined for otolaryngologic problems. Bony exostoses manifest as a gradual narrowing of the bony canal by broad-based mounds of bone that arise from the anterior and posterior canal walls.

- They usually occur in individuals with a history of cold-water exposure (such as swimmers or surfers).
- They usually occur bilaterally and are generally asymptomatic.
- Symptoms such as conductive hearing loss and otitis externa can arise if the canal becomes occluded.
- Histologic findings include a dense, stratified arrangement of new bone that is remodeled over time into normal lamellar bone.

Treatment
Surgery is indicated if the patient becomes symptomatic. A canalplasty is usually performed.

Osteoma

An osteoma manifests as a discrete, pedunculated bony mass that arises from the tympanosquamous suture line adjacent to the bony–cartilaginous junction.

- It is usually solitary and unilateral.
- These are the most common bony neoplasms of the external ear canal
- Like exostoses, osteomas are usually asymptomatic; however, symptoms can arise if canal obstruction occurs.
- No link to cold-water exposure or radiation has been demonstrated.
- Histology reveals well-formed lamellae with multiple fibrovascular channels throughout the interlamellar spaces.

Treatment is similar to that for exostoses.

Relapsing polychondritis

This is an autoimmune disorder in which an individual exhibits a systemic destruction of articular and nonarticular cartilage. It characteristically affects the head and neck (e.g., eyes, ears, eustachian tube, nose), respiratory system (e.g., larynx, trachea, bronchi), cardiovascular system (e.g., heart valves, blood vessels), and joints. The external ear is affected in almost 90% of cases. Auricular signs and systems affected:

- Recurrent cellulitis of one or both pinna. The earlobes are typically spared.
- Destruction of EAC cartilage may result in conductive hearing loss.

Treatment is with systemic corticosteroids, NSAIDs, or colchicines.

Ramsay Hunt syndrome

Also known as herpes zoster oticus, this syndrome is caused by varicella-zoster viral infection. It has the following symptoms:

- Facial nerve paralysis
- Sensorineural hearing loss
- Bullous myringitis and a vesicular eruption of the concha of the pinna and the EAC

Treatment includes use of an antiviral agent (e.g., valacyclovir) and systemic steroids.

The middle ear

Structure and function

The middle ear is made up of the following structures (see p. 235, Fig. 12.2):

- Tympanic membrane
- Ossicular chain
- Nerves of the middle ear
- Muscles of the middle ear
- Mastoid air cell system
- Eustachian tube

The function of the middle ear is to transduce sound waves, amplify them, and pass them to the cochlea. There is also an intrinsic mechanism to protect the ear from loud noise.

Tympanic membrane

The tympanic membrane (Fig. 13.1) is composed of three layers. It is divided into the pars flaccida and the pars tensa by the anterior and posterior malleolar folds. These two parts differ in their strength. The pars tensa has collagen fibers arranged radially, and the flaccida has randomly arranged collagen and a high elastin content. The squamous epithelium grows from central drum germinal centers. It then migrates radially and out along the external auditory canal (EAC) to be shed at the external auditory meatus (EAM).

The ossicular chain

The malleus, incus, and stapes conduct and amplify sound. The difference in contact area between the drum and the malleus compared to the contact area between the stapes and the oval window leads to an amplification. When this is added to the mechanical advantage of the articulated ossicular chain, the total amplification is in the order of 22 times.

Nerves of the middle ear

The facial nerve has an intricate course. The chorda tympani is a branch of the facial nerve. The tympanic plexus has secretomotor fibers to the parotid. (see Fig. 13.2)

Muscles of the middle ear

The stapedius contracts and damps the movement of stapes. The tensor tympani contracts and stabilizes the movement of the malleus. Both of these mechanisms protect the ear from loud noise.

Mastoid air cell system

This connects with the middle ear via the antrum. It provides a reservoir of air to balance vast changes in air pressure.

Eustachian tube

This tube provides a mechanism for the equalization of air pressure on either side of the eardrum.

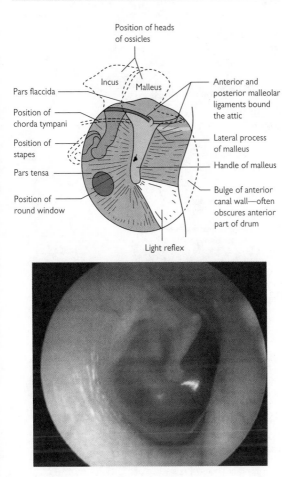

Position of heads of ossicles

Incus   Malleus

Pars flaccida

Position of chorda tympani

Position of stapes

Pars tensa

Position of round window

Anterior and posterior malleolar ligaments bound the attic

Lateral process of malleus

Handle of malleus

Bulge of anterior canal wall—often obscures anterior part of drum

Light reflex

Fig. 13.1 Diagram of tympanic membrane showing quadrants and what lies behind.

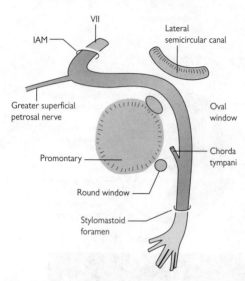

Fig. 13.2 The medial wall of the middle ear.

Congenital abnormalities

Congenital abnormalities of the middle ear are rare in isolation. Middle ear abnormalities are more common in association with microtia (see p. 236). Abnormalities of the ossicular chain can occur in isolation.

Signs and symptoms
- Conductive hearing loss is never more than 60 dB.
- Normal tympanogram/As type/Ad type.

Management
- Diagnosis is usually suggested on CT and confirmed by performing a tympanotomy.
- If the abnormality is in the better hearing ear, use a hearing aid. Surgery carries a higher risk of permanent sensorineural loss.
- If the abnormality is in the worse hearing ear, then consider a tympanotomy after a trial of a hearing aid.

Acute otitis media

This is a very common condition (see Fig. 13.3). Almost everyone will suffer with acute otitis media during their lifetime. Signs and symptoms may include a preceding URTI, severe and progressive otalgia, or a discharge—this is usually associated with a resolution of the otalgia. A diagnosis is made by taking a history, examining the tympanic membrane, and taking the patient's temperature.

Treatment for acute otitis media is controversial. Systematic review suggests treatment with analgesia only. However, these reviews may have included a high proportion of viral ear infections, for which antibiotics would not be expected to be useful.

Management
- Give analgesia in all cases.
- Give oral antibiotics for 1 week.
- Discharge may continue for 1 week.
- When infection has resolved, always check that the tympanic membrane is normal.

Recurrent infections of the middle ear
These must be differentiated from one persisting infection. Treat any acute infection actively as above. If the patient has more than five infections in 6 months, then consider alternative treatment.

Treatment
- Medical—consider prophylactic therapy.
- Surgical—if there is effusion or glue ear consider grommet insertion ± adenoidectomy.
- All treatment needs monitoring—use an infection diary to record episodes of infection pre- and post-treatment.

Caution
Acute otitis media is often misdiagnosed. Children with nocturnal earache often have glue ear or eustachian tube dysfunction. The tympanic membrane may be red or injected, but there is no discharge and the pain resolves very quickly upon waking.

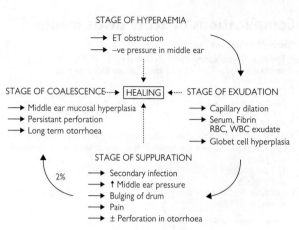

Fig. 13.3 Diagram of stages of acute otitis media.

Complications of acute otitis media

Chronic infection

- The infection may persist and become chronic. This may be due to resistant bacteria. Use a broad-spectrum antibiotic such as Ciprofloxacin.
- Consider myringotomy for relief of symptoms or to obtain microbiological information.

Facial nerve palsy

- Ten percent of people have a dehiscent facial nerve when the bony covering is absent over the nerve. This results in facial nerve irritation and palsy.
- The patient must be admitted to the hospital and given IV antibiotics and steroids.
- Consider myringotomy and grommet insertion if the condition fails to resolve in 24 hours.

Acute mastoiditis

This is an infection of the mastoid air cells that will lead to a severe earache with tenderness, swelling and redness behind the pinna. The pinna may also be pushed forward, making it look more prominent.

This is an ENT emergency and requires admission and IV antibiotics and possible surgical drainage.

Perforation of tympanic membrane

Repeated infections that perforate the tympanic membrane can lead to perforations that do not heal.

Sensorineural hearing loss (SNHL)

Rarely, toxins can spread to the inner ear to produce a sensorineural hearing loss. This is a greater risk with recurrent infection.

Vertigo

Infection near the lateral semicircular canal can produce a para labynthitis. This can cause a spectrum of vestibular disturbance ranging from mild unsteadiness to disabling vertigo.

Glue ear

Glue ear is caused by a combination of exposure to infection and a non-functioning eustachian tube. Almost 8 out of 10 children will have glue ear at some time during childhood. The incidence of glue ear decreases with age as the immune system develops and the eustachian tube becomes larger.

The signs and symptoms of glue ear can include decreased hearing, recurrent ear infections, poor speech development, failing performance at school and, sometimes, antisocial behavior.

Risk factors
- Smoking parents
- Bottle feeding
- Day-care nursery
- Cleft palate
- Atopy

Investigations

Take a full history, do a full examination including the palate, and carry out age-appropriate audiometry (see p. 70) and tympanometry.

Management

This depends on a balance of the following:
- *Social factors*—more urgent action is needed if the family is unlikely to make it to further appointments.
- *Hearing disability*—how the child is coping with their hearing problem socially and at school is more important than the actual level of hearing loss.
- *Appearance of tympanic membranes*—if there is gross retraction, intervention may be needed to avoid retraction pocket formation.

Treatment

There are three options:
- *Watchful waiting*—this should apply to all patients for 3 months, as glue ear will resolve in 50% of cases.
- *Hearing aid*—there is a window of opportunity at 4–8 years old. It is noninvasive, but may lead to teasing at school.
- *Insertion of grommets*—short general anesthetic (GA) and adenoidectomy—see p. 366.

Chronic suppurative otitis media without cholesteatoma

This common condition is associated with eustachian tube dysfunction with or without an infection in the mastoid. As with other ear diseases, its prevalence continues despite antibiotics.

The signs and symptoms of chronic suppurative otitis media include continuous recurrent otorrhea, perforation in tympanic membrane (Fig. 13.4, usually central), and no cholesteatoma present.

Risk factors
- Smoking patient
- Smoking parents
- Acute otitis media
- Decreased immunity

Investigations
- Take a full history and do an ENT examination.
- Do a microscopy of the eardrum with thorough cleaning.
- Take a swab for microbiology.

Management
- Give appropriate topical and systemic antibiotics based on the swab result. The condition may settle with antibiotics and water precautions.
- Perform a regular aural toilet.
- Persistent infections may need surgery in the form of myringoplasty and mastoidectomy.

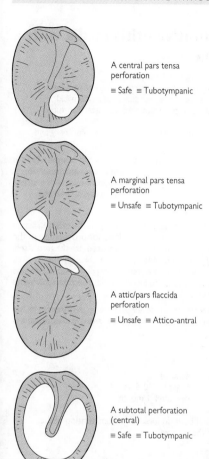

A central pars tensa perforation

≡ Safe ≡ Tubotympanic

A marginal pars tensa perforation

≡ Unsafe ≡ Tubotympanic

A attic/pars flaccida perforation

≡ Unsafe ≡ Attico-antral

A subtotal perforation (central)

≡ Safe ≡ Tubotympanic

Fig. 13.4 Diagram showing sites of perforations. Safe/unsafe refers to the risk of developing an associated cholesteatoma.

Chronic suppurative otitis media with cholesteatoma

This is often divided into congenital and acquired:
- **Congenital cholesteatoma** results from an abnormal focus of squamous epithelium in the middle ear space, i.e., a dermoid.
- **Acquired cholesteatoma** results from chronic eustachian tube dysfunction.
  - Acquired cholesteatoma is further subdivided into primary and secondary forms.

It was hoped that the incidence of this condition would change with the advent of antibiotics. Unfortunately, the disease continues, presenting at any age. Signs and symptoms include recurrent otitis media with a smelly mucopurulent discharge, hearing loss, facial nerve palsy, and vertigo.

Development of a cholesteatoma

Primary acquired cholesteatoma develops from a pars flaccida retraction pocket. Prolonged low middle-ear pressure allows for propagation of the pocket. The pocket neck becomes small compared to the sac itself. Initially, squamous epithelium migrates with ease through the pocket. As the sac gets bigger the squamous epithelium builds up inside the pocket. Eventually germinal centers are incorporated. Infection supervenes on the impacted squamous epithelium/keratin.

Secondary acquired cholesteatoma develops from a perforation in the pars tensa. Epithelium then invades the middle ear and a cholesteatoma is formed.

Investigations
- Aural toilet
- Microscopy and suction clearance
- Topical antibiotic/steroid drops for 10 days
- Review under the microscope after 1 month
- Audiometry
- CT scan of the temporal bone to look for pneumatization of the mastoid or erosion of the scutum.

Management

This depends on the age and fitness of the patient, which ear is affected, the patient's wishes, and their ability to tolerate ear toilet.

Prophylaxis This is a controversial treatment in which early retraction pockets are treated by inserting a grommet to reverse the development of a cholesteatoma.

Early retraction pocket Attempt to clean the pocket and remove keratin. GA may be required. Maintenance of a cleaned pocket can be undertaken with regular aural toilet.

Established non-cleaning pocket If the worse hearing ear is affected, surgery will be required to remove the risk of intracerebral complications. See Mastoid surgery, p. 266.

Follow-up

These patients are at risk of recurrence and need careful follow-up.

Mastoid surgery

Cortical mastoidectomy

A simple opening of the mastoid and ablation of the individual air cell are performed to create one large cavity or drain pus. This procedure was frequently performed in the pre-antibiotic ear to treat acute mastoiditis, but is now much less common and usually performed as part of a more complicated mastoid operation.

Modified radical mastoidectomy (MRM)

See Fig. 13.5. This is performed to remove cholesteatoma from the middle ear and mastoid. The cholesteatoma, head of the malleus, and incus are all removed and the connections between the middle ear cleft and mastoid are enlarged. A "mastoid cavity" is created by removal of the posterior canal wall; this may require cleaning in outpatients.

Combined approach tympanoplasty (CAT) (canal wall-up mastoidectomy)

This operation is also performed for cholesteatoma, but here the posterior canal wall remains intact and no cavity is formed. The eardrum looks normal after the operation. Benefits of this approach include less outpatient care, better hearing results, and patients being better able to tolerate swimming. However, since cholesteatoma can be "sealed in" behind an intact drum, a "second-look" operation is required at 6–12 months to ensure that the disease has been eradicated.

(a)　　　　　　　　　　　　　　　(b)

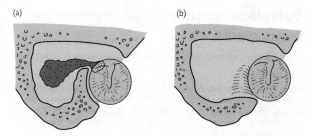

Fig. 13.5 (a) An attic cholesteatoma extending backward into the mastoid.
(b) Modified radical mastoidectomy. Here the cholesteatoma has been removed and
the mastoid cavity "exteriorized," i.e., connected to the ear canal by removal of the
posterior ear canal wall.

Complications of chronic suppurative otitis media

These are related to local and distant effects of cholesteatoma (see Fig. 13.6).

Local effects

Conductive hearing loss Because the retracted attic segment of the eardrum lies against the long process of the eardrum, it interferes with its already tenuous blood supply. The incus initially thins, then loses its attachment to the stapes. The cholesteatoma can bridge this gap and temporarily improve the conductive loss.

Sensorineural hearing loss The toxic effect of the local infection can cause a sensorineural hearing loss.

Vertigo may be due to a paralabrynthitis causing an irritative vestibulopathy, or it may be the result of erosion into the lateral semicircular canal, called a fistula.

Facial nerve dysfunction If a dehiscence exists, infection can produce direct irritation of the nerve. The cholesteatoma may also directly erode the bony covering of the facial nerve.

Mastoiditis A chronic infection may lead to mastoiditis.

Distant effects

Meningitis The roof of the middle ear is also the floor of the middle cranial fossa. A thin plate of bone separates the middle ear from the meninges in this area. This can be eroded by an extensive cholesteatoma, with a spread of infection to the meninges.

Cerebral abscess A spread of infection can lead to abscess formation, which can progress to the temporal lobe.

Lateral sinus thrombosis The lateral sinus is one of the relations of the mastoid air cell systems. Infection can spread to the lateral sinus, causing local thrombosis. This in turn can lead to hydrocephalus.

Bezolds abscess Infection from the mastoid spreads through the mastoid tip and travels under the sternocleidomastoid muscle. It then points in the neck anterior to the muscle.

Citellis abscess Infection spreads medially from the mastoid tip to collect in the digastric fossa.

① Mastoiditis
② Labyrinthitis
③ Extracliral abscess
④ Sigmoid sinus thrombosis
⑤ Temperal lobe abscess
⑥ Meningitis

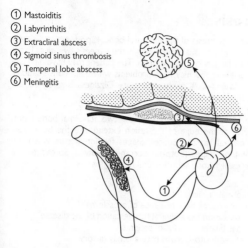

Fig. 13.6 Routes of spread of infection from the middle ear.

Otosclerosis

This is an osseous dyscrasia of the temporal bone. It presents as a slowly progressive hearing loss, usually beginning in the patient's twenties. There is usually a family history of the condition. The patient may have difficulty hearing when chewing and may have problems with quiet conversations. Tinnitus occurs in 69%–80% of these patients. Dizziness is rarely caused by this condition. There is no history of infection.

In its early stages the lesion is "spongiotic." Later, this spongiosis becomes sclerosis or a combination of these two abnormal bone types. Later, osteocytes at the edge of the lesion extend into the bone, surrounding the central vascular spaces. Stapes fixation occurs when the annular ligament or stapes footplate becomes involved. Spread to the cochlea produces high-tone sensorineural hearing loss.

Incidence

- The female-to-male ratio is 2 to 1.
- 6.4% of temporal bones have evidence of otosclerosis.
- 0.3% of the population has a clinical manifestation of the disease.
- The condition is bilateral in 70% of patients.
- 50% of patients with otosclerosis have a family history.

Investigations

- Check for a normal mobile, intact tympanic membrane.
- Look for "Schwartzes sign"—a flamingo pink blush anterior to the oval window. This means there is increased vascular supply to the otospongiotic focus.
- Perform pure tone audiometry. This shows conductive hearing loss (CHL) typical of a Carhart's notch (see Fig. 13.7).
- Check for absent stapedial reflex.
- Carry out a CT scan—this may help to exclude other bony abnormalities of the middle ear such as ossicular fixation.

Differential diagnosis

Paget's disease There is other bony involvement (e.g., frontal bossing), increased alkaline phosphatase, and mixed hearing loss.

Osteogenesis imperfecta Also known as Van der Hoeve syndrome, this condition leads to mixed hearing loss with blue sclera. There is frequently a history of multiple bony fractures.

Treatment

The options are as follows:
- No treatment
- Hearing aid
- Surgery—stapedectomy after a 3-month trial of hearing aid

Contra-indications to surgery

- Surgery should be performed on a worse-hearing ear only.
- Previous sensorineural hearing loss in contralateral ear.
- If there is tympanic membrane perforation, this will necessitate a myringoplasty first.
- Infection.

Cochlear otosclerosis

This is due to spread of the otosclerotic process to the basal turn of the cochlea. Treatment with sodium fluoride helps to reduce the abnormal bone metabolism and thus stabilize hearing loss. Monitor with serial pure tone audiograms.

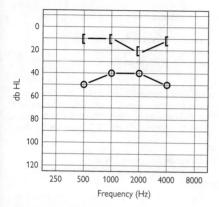

Fig. 13.7 Pure tone audiometry showing conductive hearing loss typical of Cahart's notch.

Trauma

Acoustic trauma

Loud noise can produce direct traumatic effects on the middle ear. See Chapter 14, p. 275 (noise-induced hearing loss).

Head injury

Direct blows to the head can produce:
- A temporal bone fracture—p. 324
- A coexistent hemotympanum—blood in the middle ear
- Ossicular chain disruption
- Rarely, cochlea concussion can produce an SNHL.

Management

Patients with severe trauma may present late to ENT, as they usually have more pressing priorities in their management. Treat the patient's head injury and check for a cervical spine injury. Perform an otoscoopy (see Box 13.1) and look for CSF otorrhea. Check the facial nerve function.

Hearing assessment
- A tuning fork test will distinguish CHL from SNHL.
- Pure tone audiogram will confirm the tuning fork findings and will quantify any hearing defect.

Treatment

SNHL Consider steroids. Give prednisolone 1 mg/kg po 1 week if there are no contraindications. Follow with serial audiograms.

CHL No immediate treatment is required. Review as outpatient in 6 weeks. The hemotympanum will have resolved. Retest the patient's hearing. If CHL persists, check the tympanogram to ensure that there is no glue ear and consider tympanotomy with ossicular reconstruction.

Box 13.1 Pens, cotton tip applicators, and sticks

If these objects are inserted into the EAC they rarely reach the eardrum. They usually impact on the skin of the EAC and tear it, causing bleeding. Careful examination with the otoscope can usually identify this problem.

Traumatic perforations of the TM heal sponataneously. Treat hemotympanum and possible ossicular dislocation as above.

Neoplasia

Benign and malignant tumors involving the middle ear space can occur, but these are very rare.

The inner ear

Structure and function of the inner ear

The inner ear can be divided into two parts, the cochlea and the vestibular system (Fig. 14.1).

Cochlea

This is the organ of sound transduction. The cochlea is coiled as a helical form and is encased in hard bone of the petrous temporal bone. The specialized structure of the cochlea turns sound waves into electrical signals that pass to the brain.

The cochlea has a tonotopic representation—this means that different areas are frequency specific. High frequencies are dealt with at the start or at the base of the cochlea. Low tones are dealt with at the cochlea apex. See Fig. 14.2 for a cross-section of the cochlea.

The neurological pathway to the auditory cortex is best remembered by using the E COLI mnemonic: **E**ighth nerve, **C**ochlear nucleus, superior **O**live, **L**ateral lemniscus, **I**nferior colliculus.

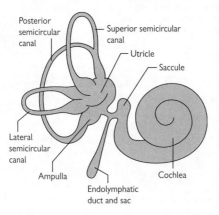

Fig. 14.1 Diagram of the inner ear.

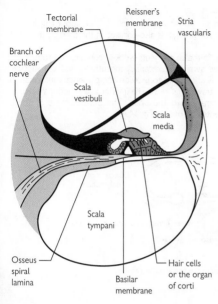

Fig. 14.2 Cross-section of the cochlea.

Vestibular system

The vestibular system functions to provide information about angular and linear acceleration for the brain. It is also encased in the petrous temporal bone.

Five separate neuroepithelial elements work in combination to provide this information: three semicircular canals, the utricle, and the saccule. The semicircular canals are paired to provide complimentary information about the direction of travel (Fig. 14.3). The inferior and superior vestibular nerves pass the information to the brain. The ultrastructure of these neuroepithelial elements is shown in Fig. 14.4.

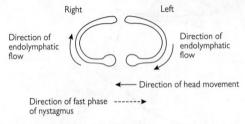

Right   Left

Direction of
endolymphatic
flow

Direction of
endolymphatic
flow

◄——— Direction of head movement

Direction of fast phase ------►
of nystagmus

Fig. 14.3 Paired motion of the semicircular canals.

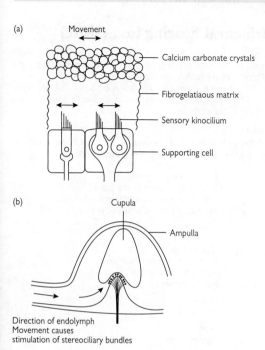

Fig. 14.4 Ultrastructure of semicircular canals and utricle.

Sensorineural hearing loss (SNHL)

The etiology of such a hearing loss can usually be determined by careful consideration of the patient's history, a clinical examination, and the findings of special investigations (see Table 14.1).

The age of onset of the patient's hearing loss is important, as is any family history of hearing loss. Careful consideration of a patient's pregnancy and perinatal history is also important.

Examination

The aim of this examination is to discover any congenital abnormality or inherited syndrome in which hearing loss may play a part.

Ears	Preauricular pits present?
	Shape and location of the pinnae
	Size of the exterior auditory canal (EAC)
	Appearance of the tympanic membrane (TM)
Eyes	Eyebrows
	Interpupillary distance
	Color of iris
	External ocular movements
	Appearance of fundus
	Retinal pigment
Face	Shape
	Symmetry
Skin	Texture
	Pigmentation
Extremities	Shape of fingers and toes
	Carrying angle

Investigations

The aim of these investigations is to confirm and assess the extent of the patient's hearing loss and to look for any evidence of an inherited condition.
- Audiological assessment
- Radiology including CT/MRI
- Blood tests including urea and electrolytes (U+E)
- Glucose
- Thyroid function test (TFT)
- EKG
- Cytogenetics

Specialist opinions

You may need to consult an ophthalmologist and/or a clinical geneticist.

Table 14.1 Classification of patients presenting with inner ear hearing loss

Nonhereditary	Hereditary
Presbyacusis	Syndromic
Noise-induced hearing loss	Non-syndromic
Idiopathic sudden hearing loss	
Autoimmune hearing loss	
Vascular causes	
Ototoxicity	
Nonorganic hearing loss	

Presbyacusis

This term describes a decreased peripheral auditory sensitivity. It is usually age related and affects men more than women.

Signs and symptoms

This condition shows itself as bilateral and progressive, with symmetrical SNHL and no history of noise exposure. The patient may have worse speech discrimination than expected on review of the audiogram. Decreasing central auditory discrimination leads to phonemic regression.

Investigations

- Otoscopy
- Pure tone audiogram (see Fig. 14.5)

Types of presbyacusis

Based on the shape of the audiogram and the site of loss, presbyacusis can be subdivided into the following subtypes:

- *Sensory presbyacusis:* steep-sloping audiogram above speech frequency. It starts in mid-life, so speech discrimination is preserved. There is degeneration in the organ of Corti.
- *Neural presbyacusis:* down-sloping high-frequency loss. Audiogram results are flatter than in sensory presbyacusis. There is thought to be first-order neuron loss, along with a disproportionate discrimination score.
- *Strial presbyacusis:* flat audiogram. There is good discrimination.
- *Cochlear conductive/indeterminate presbyacusis:* down-sloping audiogram. There is increasing stiffness of the basilar membrane.
- *Central presbyacusis* is marked by loss of GABA in the inferior colliculus
- *Middle-ear aging:* loosening of ligaments or an ossicular articulation problem occurs.

Management

The patient may be given counseling and advice about hearing loss and given a hearing aid when the symptoms are troublesome.

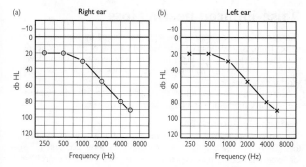

Fig. 14.5 Investigation of presbyacusis: pure tone audiogram for (a) right ear and (b) left ear.

Noise-induced hearing loss

This is defined as damage to the inner ear caused by exposure to loud noise. There is a relationship between the volume of sound and its duration that causes damage. Eight hours of exposure to a sound level of 85 dB usually causes damage. Louder sounds will cause damage at shorter exposure times.

Acoustic trauma is caused by sounds greater than 180 dB. Rupture of the tympanic membrane and ossicular fracture may occur.

Signs and symptoms

The patient will usually present with bilateral and symmetrical hearing loss. There may be a noise-induced temporary threshold shift (TTS)—for example, hearing may improve over the weekend if the problem is noise at work. The patient may have difficulty hearing in the context of background noise or they may have tinnitus.

Investigations

Use audiometry. For a typical pattern see Fig. 14.6.

Pathology

Hearing loss is greatest in the 3–6 kHz region of cochlea. Below 2 kHz the acoustic reflex is protective. EAC resonant frequency is 1–4 kHz, so energy delivered at these frequencies is greater. The actual loss of cochlea cells occurs where noise damage is greatest. Outer hair cells lose rigidity and the stereocilia fuse.

Management

Consider the following to prevent further noise damage:
• Health and safety at work
• Provision of ear plugs or muffs
• Routine hearing screening for occupations at risk

For established damage consider
• Hearing aids
• Counseling for tinnitus

▶ Rifle shooting

This will sometimes result in an asymmetric SNHL with the noise-damaged pattern. When firing a rifle, one ear is nearer to the gun barrel. If the patient shoots right-handed, their LEFT ear is most affected, as it is nearer to the barrel of the gun.

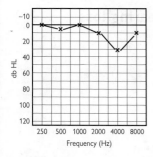

Fig. 14.6 Audiogram of presbyacusis.

Idiopathic sudden hearing loss

See Chapter 20, p. 409.

Tinnitus

This is a sensation of a noise in the ear. It can exist with a hearing loss of any cause and can even occur in patients with normal hearing. However, it is most commonly associated with sensorineural hearing loss. Most people will experience tinnitus at some time in their lives and for most it is no more than a transient nuisance. In others, however, it is a troublesome symptom that can trigger depression or even suicide. Tinnitus is usually intrinsic, i.e., only heard by the patient.

Causes of intrinsic tinnitus
- Drugs
- Labyrinthitis
- Trauma
- Vascular
- Presbycusis
- Meniere's disease
- Noise-induced hearing loss
- Otosclerosis
- Acoustic neuroma

Cause of extrinsic tinnitus
- An insect in the ear canal
- Vascular malformations
- Palatal myoclonus

The tinnitus model

Experiments have shown that 95% of normal people will experience a degree of tinnitus when put into a sound-proofed room. This means that the ear and auditory pathways are producing "noise" or electrical activity that even normally hearing people can recognize; however, our central auditory pathways filter out this useless information, and we do not normally perceive it. In fact, our CNS is constantly monitoring our surroundings, but little of this is brought to our attention. For example, up to this point you were not aware of your shoes on your feet, or the noise of passersby and traffic, but now that they have been brought to your attention you have become aware of them.

This screening system is essential to avoid sensation overload! It is believed that tinnitus becomes problematic when this screening or filtering process breaks down, and the "noise" that the ear generates is not discarded as useless information but is instead perceived as a threat, which by itself triggers an emotional reaction via the limbic system.

Tinnitus retraining therapy seeks to reverse this process by counseling the patient and removing the perception of noise as a threat (Fig. 14.7).

When meeting patients with tinnitus it is very important to avoid negative counseling such as the following: "Tinnitus—oh that's awful. I would hate to have that." Or, "Tinnitus—well there is nothing that can be done about that; you will just have to put up with it." Sentiments such as these will only serve to reinforce the negative feelings patients have about their condition and turn their feelings of "threat" into feelings of hopelessness.

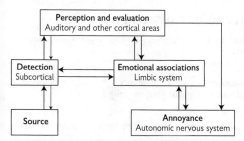

Fig. 14.7 Tinnitus retraining—diagram of model.

Autoimmune ear disease

Autoimmune ear disease is classified as either organ specific or as a systemic disease.

Organ specific

This type of disease shows vestibuloauditory autoimmunity or evidence of cell-mediated immunity against inner ear antigens.

Systemic disease

This disease type is part of a recognized systemic autoimmune disease. Common diseases that have auditory vestibular involvement are discussed below. Patients with autoimmune ear disease are usually middle-aged and are more likely to be female than male.

Signs and symptoms

- Bilateral unexplained SNHL
- May be fluctuant dizziness or Meniere's-like syndrome with aural fullness
- Rapidly progressive hearing loss over days or weeks
- Associated seventh-nerve palsy
- Normal otoscopic examination
- Coexistent systemic immune disease.

Investigations

Take a full history and give a full otoneurological examination, including a pure tone audiogram. Order an MRI scan to exclude acoustic neuroma with unilateral presentation.

Carry out the following blood tests:
- Antigen-specific antibodies
- Antigen-nonspecific antibodies
- Acute-phase reactants
- Lyme titers

Treatment

Treatment should be given under the guidance of a neurotolgist and/or a rheumatologist. Give steroids such as prednisolone 1 mg/kg per day po or give steroid-sparing alternatives:
- Cyclophosphamide
- Methotrexate
- Plasmaphoresis

The following conditions are thought to have an autoimmune basis and can cause hearing loss.

Polyarteritis nodosa

This condition affects the small and medium arteries. There is a rare association with an inner ear hearing loss.

Cogan's syndrome

This is a nonsyphilitic interstitial keratitis with vestibuloauditory dysfunction. It presents with photophobia and lacrimation 1 to 6 months before vestibuloauditory symptoms develop.

Atypical cogan's

This interstitial keratitis develops 1 to 2 years before auditory vestibular problems.

Wegener's granulomatosis

This is a necrotizing granulomatous vasculitis of the lower and upper respiratory tract that also affects the kidneys, causing focal necrotizing glomerulonephritis. Typically, 90% of patients have a sensorineural hearing loss and 20% have a conductive hearing loss with effusion. Also, 90% of patients are cANCA positive.

Relapsing polychondritis

In this condition, giant-cell arteritis and systemic vasculitis cause recurrent episodes of inflammatory necrosis. There is a raised ESR and a false positive VDRL.

Rheumatoid arthritis

This is a very common condition with characteristic arthropathy.

Ototoxicity

Because drugs can damage the cochlea and vestibular system, it is worth taking a careful drug history, as a wide range of drugs can cause symptoms. Check with the U.S. Food and Drug Administration (FDA) or the Physician's Desk Reference (PDR) for side effects.

Aminoglycoside antibiotics

These antibiotics have a narrow therapeutic index and can cause damage to the inner ear. Common side effects are drug-induced vestibular symptoms and hearing loss.

Patients requiring parenteral aminoglycoside antibiotics should have the plasma levels of the drug monitored during therapy. Local policy varies; often trough levels of antibiotic are used to determine future dose levels.

Topical antibiotics

Most topical antibiotics available contain an aminoglycoside antibiotic. These drugs are experimentally ototoxic in guinea pigs and other animals. They are believed to enter the inner ear through the round-window membrane, causing direct ototoxic effects. Drug data sheets also warn of the risks of using these preparations when there are grommets in situ or there is a perforation of the TM.

▶ Short courses of these topical antibiotics—less than 10 days—are safe for treating perforations or grommets in the presence of infection. Edema of the middle ear mucosa with a thickened round-window membrane limits the entry of antibiotic into the inner ear. *Untreated infection is a greater risk to hearing than the antibiotic.*

Therapeutic uses

Aminoglycosides can be used to treat patients with Meniere's disease by causing a vestibulopathy when instilled into the middle ear. Much higher doses are used than with the standard drops.

Other drugs

Chemotherapy, especially cisplatin, induces SNHL. Aspirin and erythromycin can cause a reversible SNHL. Patients present with tinnitus. Vancomycin and loop diuretics can also cause ototoxicity.

Hereditary hearing loss

Heredited hearing loss may be divided into syndromic and non-syndromic types. Non-syndromic or nonorganic hearing loss is most common, representing about two-thirds of cases.

As the loci of genes associated with hearing loss are identified, it becomes more obvious that the classifying of these conditions on a syndromic basis may be misleading. Many patients with apparently non-syndromic hereditary hearing loss have the same gene alterations as their syndromic counterparts but are not phenotypically syndromic.

Other classifications of hereditary hearing loss are as follows:

Genetics	See Table 14.2
Age of onset	Early (birth to age 2)
	Known congenital
	Suspected congenital
	Delayed (3–20 years)
	Adult (>21 years)
Hearing loss	Sensorineural
	Conductive
	Mixed hearing loss
Laterality	Unilateral/bilateral
Stability	Stable
	Fluctuating
	Progressive
Frequencies	Low (250 Hz–1 kHz)
	Medium (>1–4 kHz)
	High (>4 kHz)
Associations	Radiological abnormalities
	Vestibular dysfunction

Table 14.2 Genetic inheritance of hearing loss

Inheritance	Percentage	Condition
Autosomal recessive	60%–70%	Non-syndromic SNHL
		Pendred syndrome
		Usher syndrome
		Jervell and Lange-Nielsen syndrome
Autosomal dominant	20%–25%	Waardenburg syndrome
		Branchial-oto-rhenal (BOR) syndrome
		Alport syndrome
X-linked recessive	2%–3%	X-linked mixed hearing loss with stapes gusher
X-linked dominant	Uncertain	Alport syndrome
Chromosomal	<1%	
Mitochondrial	<1%	
Multifactorial	Uncertain	

Syndromic hearing loss

Goldenhaar's syndrome (oculoauricularvertebral [OAV] syndrome)

This is the most common syndrome (see Fig. 14.8), occurring in approximately 1 in 10,000 live births. It is sporadic, not caused by genetic inheritance.

Features of Goldenhaar's syndrome

Face	Marked asymmetry in 25%
	Maxilla and temporal bones reduced and flattened
	Hypoplasia/aplasia of mandible
Ear	Flattened helical rim
	Preauricular tags
	EAC atretic/small
Hearing loss	CHL
	SNHL in 15%
Associations	Skeletal abnormalities c-spine/skull base
	Cleft lip/palate
	Velopharyngeal insufficiency
	Mental retardation in 15%

Treacher–Collins syndrome

Patients have a mandibulofacial dysostosis due to first/second branchial arch, and groove and pouch abnormalities (see Fig. 14.9). This is the most common syndrome of hearing loss. Sixty percent of cases are sporadic rather than genetic. This abnormality has been found to occur on gene 5q 31–4.

Features of Treacher–Collins syndrome

Face	Depressed cheeks
	Narrow midface
	Malformed pinnae, cup shaped
	Hypertelorism
Ear	Narrow EAC
	Malformed ossicles, cochlea, and labyrinth
Associations	Cleft palate
	Palatopharyngeal incompetence in 30%–40%
	Normal intelligence

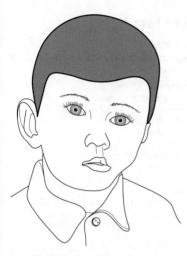

Fig. 14.8 Features of Goldenhaar's syndrome.

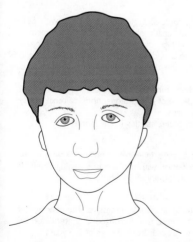

Fig. 14.9 Features of Treacher–Collins syndrome.

Syndromic hearing loss II

Waardenburg syndrome (WS)

Between 2% and 5% of congenitally deaf children have Waardenburg syndrome.

Features of Waardenburg syndrome

Appearance	Dystopia canthorum in type 1
	Synophrys—confluent eyebrows in 85% of type 1
	Heterochromia iridis (different color irides)
	Broad nasal root
	Sapphire eyes
	White forelock in 30%–40%
	Vitiligo
	Premature gray hair
Hearing loss	Congenital SNHL
	20% of those with type 1 WS and 50% of those with type 2 have a hearing loss
	50% of people with WS have normal hearing

Branchial-oto-renal (BOR) syndrome

In this rare condition there is an association of branchial fistulas or cysts with hearing problems and renal abnormalities.

Alport syndrome

This is a rare hereditary, progressive glomerulonephritis with SNHL. It presents as hearing loss and renal problems. There are six subtypes of Alport syndrome, classified by type of inheritance, age of onset of renal failure, presence of hearing loss, and ocular abnormalities. The diagnosis of Alport syndrome depends on three of the following features being found:

• Positive family history of hematuria and renal failure
• Electron-microscopic evidence of glomerulonephritis on renal biopsy
• Characteristic ophthalmic signs
• Progressive high-frequency SNHL starting in childhood

Pendred syndrome

This is a rare autosomal recessive, inherited condition in which a non-toxic goiter is found in association with profound congenital SNHL. It is associated with the mondini deformity of the cochlea.

Jervell and Lange-Nielsen syndrome

This condition is believed to be autosomal recessive. The abnormality is located on chromosome 11. There is a prolonged QT interval on EKG. Multiple syncopal episodes may occur from the age of 3–5 years on.

Usher syndrome

This is an autosomal recessive condition consisting of retinitis pigmentosa and hearing impairment.

Nonorganic hearing loss (NOHL)

This describes a situation in which a patient claims to have a hearing loss where none exists, or one in which a patient exaggerates a hearing loss that does exist.

A typical example may be a child who is having difficulties at school or at home, and who presents with a very poor hearing test result. Often the hearing loss documented on the audiogram will seem out of keeping with the child's participation in the consultation. Another example is a patient who is pursuing a claim for damages as a result of a hearing loss.

The clues to look for when diagnosing this condition are concerns raised by the audiologist about inconsistent results, litigation involvement, or unusual parent–child interaction.

Investigations

- Pure tone audiometry
- Stenger test
- Speech audiogram—it is more difficult to fabricate an abnormal response.
- Stapedial reflex testing
- Delayed speech feedback—the patient reads aloud and their speech is played into the affected ear. The playback is slightly delayed, which will cause the patient to hesitate or stutter if they can hear.
- Brainstem-evoked auditory response—this is the gold standard in litigation cases.

Management

Careful handling of nonorganic hearing loss is required. It may be wise to suggest to affected children that you know their hearing is better, but don't be too confrontational. Bring them back for another audiogram and suggest that they try to be a little more accurate.

Litigation claims need more tact and multiple investigations before undertaking any confrontation.

Stenger test

Use two 512 Hz tuning forks. This test can also be performed in the audiology booth.

Step 1

The patient closes their eyes and the examiner stands behind the patient. The tuning fork is activated and placed 5 cm from each ear in turn. The patient will hear the note in their good ear but deny hearing it in the nonhearing ear.

Step 2

Both tuning forks are used without the patient realizing it. One is held 5 cm from the ear with the alleged poor hearing. The other is held, at the same time, 15 cm away from the good ear. The patient with NOHL will deny hearing any sound. The tuning fork held near the bad ear will mask the sound of the tuning fork near the good ear. The genuine patient will only hear the tuning fork near the good ear.

Labyrinthitis (vestibular neuronitis)

This presents as a sudden episode of vertigo in a previously well person. It is equally common in men and women, with the usual age of onset being 30 to 40 years. Attacks are usually single, but people may occasionally experience multiple attacks, and it can be recurrent. It normally lasts 1–2 days and improves over weeks. Vertigo is usually unilateral or, rarely, bilateral. Epidemics can occur in the spring or summer. There may be an associated URTI 2 weeks prior to the vertigo. It occasionally leaves a BPPV symptom complex.

Pathology
- Axonal loss—endoneurial fibrosis and atrophy of the nerve
- Suspected viral etiology, e.g., rubeola, HSV, reovirus, CMV, influenza, and mumps

Investigations
- Pure tone audiograms
- Nystagmus away from affected side
- Quix test positive (seated Romberg test)
- ENG if there is clinical doubt about the diagnosis
- MRI if there is asymmetry or recurrent episodes

Treatment
- Vestibular suppressant for acute attack—Stemetil 5 mg sub-buccal/ 12.5 mg IM
- Steroids if there is SNHL—prednisolone 1 mg/kg for 1 week
- Patients usually compensate well for this condition.
- Vestibular rehabilitation for patients who do not compensate

Benign paroxysmal positional vertigo

This is the most common cause of peripheral vertigo. It usually starts around the age of 50 years. The patient experiences brief episodes of vertigo caused by changes in position, in particular looking up and rolling over in bed. It is worse in the morning and evening. This condition is believed to occur as a result of stimulation of the semicircular canals by otoliths that have become misplaced.

There are three typical patterns in benign paroxysmal positional vertigo (BPPV):

- Acute form—resolves in 3 months
- Intermittent form—active and inactive periods over years
- Chronic form—has continuous symptoms over longer duration

Investigations

- Full otoneurological examination
- Dix-Hallpike test
- Pure tone audiogram
- ENG if there is diagnostic uncertainty
- MRI scan if symptoms persist for more than 3 months

Dix-Hallpike test

Have the patient sit on the examining table positioned in such a way that when they lie back their head will be over the end of the bed. While the patient is sitting, turn their head 30° toward the examiner. This leads to maximal stimulation of the posterior semicircular canal (PSCC) on lying down. Then ask the patient to lie down and look at the examiner's nose. The examiner supports the head and allows the head to extend over the edge of the bed. A positive test results in rotatory nystagmus after a delay of 1–5 seconds. This lasts between 10 and 30 seconds. Reversal to the upright position changes the direction of the nystagmus. This process is fatigable and sensitivity of the test can be improved with Frenzel glasses, which do not allow optic fixation.

Treatment

Fatiguing exercises are used if the patient has significant symptom-free episodes (see Fig. 14.10).

Epley maneuver can bring 90% relief if the patient has had symptoms, by repositioning the displaced otoliths (see Fig. 14.11).

Surgery This is rare. A singular neurectomy may lead to SNHL in 10%–20% of patients. A retrosigmoid vestibular nerve section may result in 1% mortality, as the procedure involves craniotomy. A posterior canal occlusion via a mastoid operation will control the symptoms, but a SNHL may complicate 5% of cases.

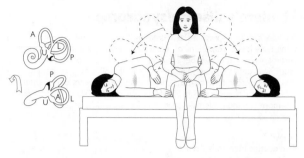

Fig. 14.10 Brandt Doroff exercises.

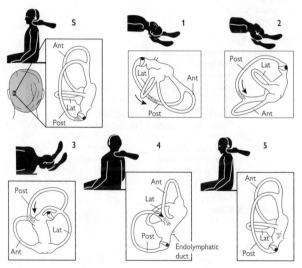

Fig. 14.11 Epley maneuver.

Meniere's disease/syndrome

Meniere's disease presents as increasing fullness in the ear and roaring tinnitus, with a sensation of blocked hearing, and episodic vertigo. Alternatively, there may be a sudden onset of vertigo with no warning (see Signs and symptoms, p. 304). Typically, 30%–50% of people with Meniere's disease have bilateral symptoms within 3 years of presentation.

Meniere's disease occurs in 50–150 people per 100,000 of the population. It is more common in females than in males and usually occurs between the ages of 35 and 40 years.

Causes
- Idiopathic Meniere's disease
- Post-traumatic head injury or ear surgery
- Postinfectious delayed, e.g., in mumps and measles
- Late-stage syphilis
- Classical Cogan's
- Atypical Cogan's

Signs and symptoms
Of people with Meniere's disease.
- 42% have hearing loss alone
- 11% have vertigo alone
- 44% have vertigo and hearing loss
- 3% have tinnitus

Vertigo lasts more than 20 minutes and is associated with nausea, vomiting, and autonomic effects. Most episodes last 2–4 hours (although some last for more than 6 hours).

Horizontal or horizontorotatory nystagmus is always present. The patient may experience *disequilibrium* after an attack for several days.

A *fluctuating SNHL* is found in the early stages of the disease. Later, the hearing loss becomes permanent. The hearing may not change for some days after an attack.

Types of hearing loss
- Low-frequency SNHL
- Flat, moderately severe SNHL
- Bilateral SNHL with >25 dB asymmetry

Poorly controlled patients have progressive hearing loss, stabilizing at 50–60 dB.

Variant presentations of Meniere's disease
- Lemoyez variant—hearing improves with vertigo attacks
- Otolithic crisis of Tumarkin—patient has drop attacks with vertigo (decompression of saccule)
- Cochlear Meniere's—auditory symptoms only
- Vestibular Meniere's—vestibular symptoms only

Investigations

There is no single diagnostic test.
- Otoneurological examination
- Pure tone audiogram
- MRI scan if there is asymmetry
- Autoantibodies—ESR, ANA, RhF, IgG
- Electrocochleography (ECoG)—this test involves placing a recording electrode either in the EAC or through the tympanic membrane to rest against the promontory of the cochlea. Sound is then applied to the test ear and the electrical activity in the ear is documented. Several components can be identified and measured. An increased ratio of the summating potential compared to the action potential >0.4 suggests hydrops (Fig. 14.12).

Pathology

On sectioning the inner ear in affected patients, the scala media is expanded, as if there has been too much pressure in the endolymph. This is known as endolymphatic hydrops.

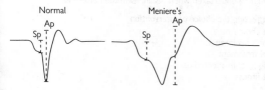

Fig. 14.12 Diagram of ECoG waveform.

Treatment of Meniere's disease

Medical management
- Prophylaxis—A low-salt diet is always recommended. A diuretic such as triamterene/hydrochlorothiazide or acetazolomide is often prescribed.
- For acute attacks of vertigo—Meclizine and promethazine are antihistamines and vestibular suppressants.
- Six-month review with symptom diary recording vertigo (spinning) episodes and the length of each episode.

Surgical intervention
Patients whose symptoms are not improved by maximum medical therapy will require active intervention.

Principles of intervention
All treatments balance the control of vertiginous episodes with the risk of hearing loss and the associated morbidity of the procedure (see Table 14.3). Treatment should not be undertaken for non-vertiginous symptoms. Care should be undertaken when dealing with the better hearing ear.

Factors affecting the choice of intervention
- Patient choice
- Surgeon's preference
- Cost of treatment
- Hearing level in affected ear
- Patient fitness

Measuring success
Guidelines from the American Academy of Otorhinolaryngologists and Head and Neck Surgeons (AAOHNS) measure success as comparing the number of vertiginous episodes in 6 months prior to treatment with the number of episodes 6 months after treatment and followed up for 2 years.

Table 14.3 Interventional treatments for Meniere's disease

Procedure	Indications	Control of vertigo	Hearing loss	Cost	Risk
Transtympanic gentamicin injection	Hearing loss <50 dB	85%	5%	Low	Low
Endolymphatic sac decompression	Fluctuating SNHL	65%	<5%	Medium	Low
Total labrynthectomy	Hearing loss >60 dB	95%	Total loss	Medium	Low–medium
Vestibular nerve section	Long-standing disease Hearing loss <50 dB	90%	<5%	High	Medium

Vascular causes of inner ear dysfunction

Vascular occlusion of the labyrinthine artery can cause the sudden onset of vertigo and hearing loss. This occlusion leads to widespread necrosis of membranous structures and labyrinthitis ossificans. The patient may have a prior history of transient ischemic attacks (TIAs)—62% of TIA patients have episodic vertigo. Compensation usually occurs in 4–6 months.

Occlusion of anterior vestibular artery

This produces hearing loss and vertigo. As the posterior circulation remains intact, the patient may simply present with a BPPV-like symptom complex.

Recurrent vestibulopathy/vascular loop syndrome

Seven percent of patients with vertigo experience this syndrome. It is believed to occur as a result of an abnormally placed blood vessel impacting on the vestibular nerve in the internal auditory meatus.

Females with this syndrome outnumber males by a 2:1 ratio. The usual age is 35–55 years old. Patients have usually had symptoms of episodic vertigo for 3 years at presentation, with 80% having had episodic vertigo within the previous year and 10% having BPPV. PTA high-frequency loss is found in 50% of patients and a middle frequency loss in 20%. The resulting histological abnormality is axonal loss and endoneurial fibrosis.

Investigations

• Full neurotological examination
• Spontaneous nystagmus
• Nonclassical Dix Hall Pike test—no fatigue
• Pure tone audiograms
• MRI/MRA

Treatment

Treatment is with vestibular suppressants—perchlorperazine or meclizine for vertigo. Also consider microvascular nerve decompression.

The skull base

Overview

The skull base is a specialized area of clinical work. No other anatomical region of the body involves such a complex proximity of neurovascular structures. Because of the rich network of blood vessels and cranial nerves, and the proximity to the brain and intracranial tissues, the surgeon must operate with tremendous care to avoid significant morbidity. The otolaryngologist is actively involved in this area, often as part of a team including a neurosurgeon or plastic or craniofacial surgeon.

Cranial-base surgery has evolved into a unique specialty of highly trained physicians. The morbidity of surgical procedures in this area has decreased secondary to improved techniques, enhanced pre- and intra-operative monitoring, and reconstructive efforts. Access to these difficult areas has increased with the development of image guidance systems and the ability to extend endoscopic sinus surgery approaches via the sphenoid and ethmoid roof to the skull base.

Anatomic considerations

Skull base regions

See Fig. 15.1.

Anterior skull base

- It extends from the frontal bone, over the cribriform plate, fovea ethmoidalis, and orbital roofs, to the greater wing of the sphenoid bone.
- The olfactory nerve (CN I) passes through foramina within the cribriform plate to the superior nasal cavity.
- The most common location of iatrogenic injury during ethmoidal surgery is at the fovea ethmoidalis.

Middle skull base

- It extends from the greater wing and body of the sphenoid bone to the petrous ridge of the temporal bone.
- Cranial nerves II through VI, the internal carotid and middle meningeal arteries, and superior ophthalmic vein traverse through foramina.
- Inferior to the skull base lie the pterygopalatine, temporal, infratemporal, and post-styloid parapharyngeal spaces.

Posterior skull base

- This extends from the petrous ridge to the occipital bones.
- It contains foramina for the jugular vein, and cranial nerves VII through XII.
- It includes the foramen magnum.
- It has grooves for the petrous, sigmoid, and transverse sinuses.

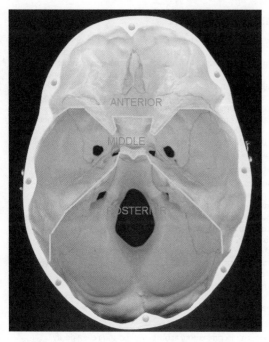

Fig. 15.1 Skull base viewed from the cranial aspect. Shown are anterior, middle, and posterior cranial fossae.

Acoustic neuroma

Acoustic neuromas are benign, slow-growing tumors derived from Schwann cells. More appropriately termed vestibular schwannomas, these tumors often originate from the vestibular nerve within the internal auditory canal (IAC). Postmortem data suggest that this tumor may be underdiagnosed. An acoustic neuroma may be found incidentally on MRI, in part because of increased detection of small tumors. See Box 15.1 for differential diagnosis of CPA angle tumors.

Acoustic neuromas account for 6%–8% of all intracranial neoplasms, most of which are sporadic (95%). Five percent of them are genetic, as part of the inherited condition of neurofibromatosis type 2 (NF2) on chromosome 22, and arise bilaterally.

Presentation

The patient may experience some of the following:
- Asymmetric sudden SNHL, progressive high-frequency SNHL, or tinnitus
- Vestibular symptoms—either disequilibrium or vertiginous episodes.
- Symptoms of raised intracranial pressure such as headache or visual disturbance.
- Brainstem compression—incoordination or ataxia gait
- Hitselberger's sign—postauricular numbness due to facial nerve compression
- Reduced corneal reflex
- Unterberger's test is positive—the patient marches on the spot with the eyes closed. A positive test is a rotation to one side or the other.

Investigations

- PTA, speech discrimination, acoustic reflex, and reflex decay
- Auditory brainstem-evoked response (ABR)
- Vestibular testing (ENG or posturography)
- MRI scan with gadolinium contrast
- Full otoneurological exam

Management

In weighing options for managing these tumors you must balance the risks of hearing loss, facial nerve palsy, and surgical morbidity. There are several possibilities:
- Observation—with serial MRI scans for slow-growing tumors
- Translabyrinthine approach—destroys the hearing but is a more direct approach. Its advantages are a low risk to the facial nerve and the ability to address larger tumor sizes.
- Middle fossa approach—technically challenging to work around the facial nerve. For small tumors only. Its advantage is improved hearing preservation.
- Retrosigmoid approach—good visualization, preserves the hearing, most tumor sizes are treatable. There is a risk of air embolism.
- Stereotactic radiosurgery—multiplanar radiotherapy, useful in treating small tumors in patients at risk for surgical resection. Its success is determined by inhibition of tumor growth.

Complications

- Any intracranial procedure, e.g., craniotomy—carries a 1% risk of mortality
- Facial nerve palsy
- Total hearing loss
- CSF leak, meningitis, air embolism, intracranial hemorrhage

---

Box 15.1 Differential diagnosis of cerebellopontine angle (CPA) tumor

- Acoustic neuroma 80%
- Meningioma
- Epidermoid cyst
- Cholesterol granuloma
- Arachnoid cyst
- Posterior cerebellar artery (PCA) aneurysm

Glomus jugulare tumors

Glomus jugulare tumors are benign paragangliomas arising from neuro-endocrine tissue (glomus bodies) within the jugular foramen. Histologically, these tumors resemble paragangliomata of the carotid body, promontory of the cochlea and adrenal medulla. Neurosecretory chief cells are arranged in nests (zellballen) surrounded by fibrous trabeculae and sustentacular cells. In contrast to secretory pheochromocytomas, only 1%–3% of glomus tumors secrete catecholamines and dopamine. Growth usually occurs through foramina and air cells but can erode bone with increasing size.

Presentation

- Asymptomatic until tumor reaches significant size
- Catecholamine excess, flushing, diarrhea, hypertension, headaches
- Compression of neurovascular structures within the jugular bulb may cause neuropathies of CN IX–XI (Vernet syndrome: paralysis of the ipsilateral soft palate, pharynx, and vocal fold).
- Petrous carotid extension may herald Horner syndrome.
- Extension to middle ear, pulsatile tinnitus, conductive hearing loss, facial weakness
- Posterior fossa extension, ataxia, and gait disturbance

Investigation

Like paragangliomas of other head and neck regions, the diagnosis of glomus jugulare tumors is facilitated through clinical exam and imaging rather than biopsy. Diagnostic biopsy is generally contraindicated because of the vascular nature of the tumors and poor accessibility.

Identification can be facilitated by the following:

- Cranial nerve and audiometric examinations
- CT scanning of temporal bone or neck with contrast delineates bony landmarks and erosion.
- MRI T1-weighted images allow determination of soft tissue and intracranial extension. Gadolinium enhancement reveals characteristic "salt and pepper" appearance of vascular channels.
- Angiography may be used to identify the vascular supply of tumor and for embolization within 48 hours of planned surgical resection.
- Consider serum catecholamine and 24-hour urinary vanillylmandellic acid and metanephrine.

Management

- Complete surgical resection is preferred.
  - Staging assists in determination of the most appropriate approach.
  - Transcervical, transmastoid, and transcranial approaches may be necessary.
- Preoperative angiography with embolization 1–2 days prior
- α- and β-blockade preoperatively if tumor is secreting
- External beam radiotherapy is considered for nonsurgical candidates but is not curative.
- Postsurgical rehabilitation for neuropathies

Nasopharyngeal carcinoma (NPC)

Because of the proximity of the nasopharynx to the skull base and vital structures, the invasive nature of tumor growth, and the difficulty of examining the region, NPC generally has a poor prognosis. There are three distinct types of nasopharyngeal carcinoma:

- Type I—keratinizing SCC. This type accounts for 25% of NPC in North American cultures, and patients at risk are similar to those with SCC of the head and neck in general.
- Type II—non-keratinizing SCC, least frequently encountered
- Type III—undifferentiated carcinoma (lymphoepithelioma). This is more common in patients from southern China and Hong Kong. It is associated with Epstein–Barr virus (EBV) and accounts for 60% of NPC in North America. Staging schema is illustrated in Box 15.2.

Presentation

- Lymph node metastasis
- Nasal obstruction
- Middle ear effusion
- Epistaxis
- Extensive tumors can involve the skull base and cause cranial nerve palsies (CN V/VI early, III/IV with cavernous sinus extension, IX/X/XI with jugular foramen involvement).

Investigations

- Thorough head and neck examination with flexible endoscopy (see Fig. 15.2).
- Patients will be given a CT and/or an MRI scan.
- FNA of involved cervical neck nodes

Important

Every patient presenting with a unilateral middle ear effusion must have their nasopharynx visualized to exclude NPC.

Treatment

- Primary treatment involves radiotherapy to the nasopharynx and bilateral neck.
- Concurrent chemoradiation may improve disease-free survival in patients with advanced disease.
- Neck dissection may be necessary if there are extensive lymph node metastases.
- Surgical treatment of NPC primary is limited by poor exposure and cranial nerve morbidity.

Prognosis

Overall prognosis is poor, with 5-year survival ranging from 30% to 57%.

Box 15.2 TNM staging of nasopharyngeal carcinoma

Primary tumor (T stage)
- T1 Tumor is confined to the nasopharynx.
- T2 Tumor extends to soft tissues of the oropharynx and/or nasal fossa.
  - T2a Without parapharyngeal extension
  - T2b With parapharyngeal extension
- T3 Tumor invades bony structures and/or paranasal sinuses
- T4 Tumor with intracranial extension and/or involvement of cranial nerves, infratemporal fossa, hypopharynx, or orbit

Lymph node metastasis (N stage)
- N0 No regional nodal metastasis
- N1 Unilateral metastasis, 6 cm or less in greatest dimension, above supraclavicular fossa
- N2 Bilateral metastasis, 6 cm or less in greatest dimension, above supraclavicular fossa
- N3a Metastasis is greater than 6 cm in dimension
- N3b Extension to the supraclavicular fossa

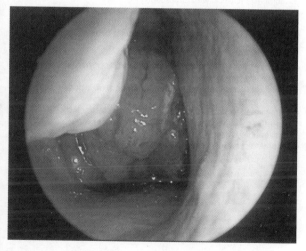

Fig. 15.2 Nasopharyngeal tumor viewed endoscopically through the nose.

Juvenile angiofibroma

This is a rare benign tumor seen almost exclusively in males. (If the patient is female, consider chromosomal analysis.) It originates near the sphenopalatine foramen at the lateral nasal wall. It may invade locally to the pterygopalatine fossa, orbit, or intracranial region but is not malignant. The histological architecture demonstrates multiple endothelial-lined vascular channels within a fibrous connective tissue stroma. The feeding vessels are often derived from the external carotid system, i.e., internal maxillary artery, but may originate from the internal carotid artery.

Presentation
- Recurrent epistaxis in young male (average age, 14 years)
- Nasal obstruction
- Unilateral middle ear effusion
- Cheek swelling
- Sinusitis
- Large posterior nasal mass
- Pulsatile mass palpated prior to adenoidectomy

Investigations
- Clinical examination with endoscope
- CT scan (bulging of the posterior maxillary sinus wall) and MRI
- Angiography
- *Do not* do a biopsy for fear of life-threatening hemorrhage

Management
- The primary treatment involves preoperative angiographic embolization followed by surgical resection 48–72 hours later.
- There are several ways to gain access to the area, including medial maxillectomy and transpalatal and midfacial degloving approaches.
- Complete resection of the tumor is facilitated by the increased exposure gained by a combined approach, such as transpalatal and midfacial degloving.
- In some cases, an endoscopic resection may be appropriate.

Sinonasal malignancy

This term describes a diverse group of malignant tumors affecting the nose and sinus system. SCC accounts for 70% of sinonasal malignancy, adenocarcinoma for 10%, and adenoid cystic carcinoma for 10%. The remainder consists of soft tissue sarcomas, lymphoreticular tumors, olfactory neuroblastoma, melanoma, and metastatic tumors. Because of the inaccessibility of the region and lack of symptoms, early diagnosis is uncommon.

Exposure to a number of industrial chemicals has been correlated with sinonasal tumors. Nickel workers are at risk of developing SCC and woodworkers are at risk for adenocarcinoma. Presentation is often delayed for up to 20 years following exposure. See Box 15.3 for staging guidelines. The overall prognosis is poor, with less than 50% of patients surviving for 5 years.

Common sites for sinonasal malignancy are the following:
- Maxillary sinus
- Nasal cavity
- Ethmoid sinus

Presentation
Some or all of the following features may be seen:
- Nasal obstruction
- Epistaxis
- Sinusitis
- Maxillary symptoms
  - Loose teeth
  - Ulcer on palate
  - Cheek swelling or hypoesthesia (infraorbital nerve involvement V2)
- Ethmoid symptoms
  - Unilateral obstruction
  - Diplopia, proptosis, chemosis
  - Headache

Investigations
- CT and/or MRI
- Endoscopy and biopsy (see Fig. 15.3)
- FNA if cervical metastases

Treatment
Because of the advanced stage of disease at diagnosis, most tumors are treated with combined surgical resection and radiotherapy. The location and extent of disease dictate the extent and approach of surgery. Localized tumors of the maxillary sinus require maxillectomy. An attempt is made to preserve the orbit when possible. Advanced tumors of the frontal, ethmoid, and sphenoid sinuses with involvement of the skull base often require craniofacial resection with neurosurgery. Rehabilitation following surgery may be improved with the use of prothodontics or flap reconstruction.

Box 15.3 TNM Staging of sinonasal malignancy

Maxillary sinus

- T1   Tumor limited to antral mucosa
- T2   Tumor causing erosion or destruction of bone into hard palate or lateral nasal wall
- T3   Tumor eroding posterior wall, subcutaneous layer, cheek, floor or medial wall of orbit, pterygoid fossa, or ethmoid sinus
- T4a   Involves anterior orbit, skin of cheek, pterygoid plates, infratemporal fossa, cribriform plate, sphenoid, frontal sinus
- T4b   Involves orbital apex, dura, brain, middle cranial fossa, cranial nerves, nasopharynx, clivus

Ethmoid sinus

- T1   Confined to ethmoid
- T2   Extends to nasal cavity or other region of nasoethmoid
- T3   Extends to medial wall or floor of orbit, maxillary sinus, palate
- T4a   Involves anterior orbit, skin of cheek, pterygoid plates, infratemporal fossa, cribriform plate, sphenoid, frontal sinus
- T4b   Involves orbital apex, dura, brain, middle cranial fossa, cranial nerves, nasopharynx, clivus

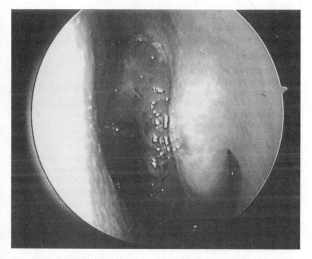

Fig. 15.3 Endoscopic view of sinonasal tumor originating from left middle meatus.

Temporal bone fractures

Fractures of the temporal bone may occur following significant blunt or penetrating trauma to the head. Etiologies include missile, thermal, blast, foreign body, or blunt head injury. Fistfights, falls, motor vehicle, and machinery accidents account for most cases. It is crucial to perform a thorough initial evaluation (airway, breathing, circulation [ABC]) and rule out coexistent trauma such as spinal, brain, thoracic, and abdominal injury.

Classically, fractures have been described by the direction of the fracture line along the petrous ridge (see Figs. 15.4 and 15.5). Longitudinal fractures (80% of total) occur following temporal or parietal blows, through foramina anterior to the ridge. Look for ruptured tympanic membrane (TM), hemotympanum, conductive hearing loss, and Battle's sign (mastoid ecchymosis). Transverse fractures (10% of total) occur from frontal or occipital blows and cross the otic capsule or IAC, imparting significant long-term morbidity. There is a higher incidence of facial-nerve and cochleovestibular injury.

Presentation
- TM laceration, EAC fracture or laceration, mastoid ecchymosis
- Hemotympanum
- Conductive or sensorineural hearing loss
- Acute vertigo
- Facial paralysis or paresis
- CSF otorrhea

Investigations
- Otoscopic evaluation
- Cranial nerve exam
- High-resolution CT temporal bone
- Tuning fork evaluation or complete audiometry
- β_2-transferrin assay for ear fluid (if applicable)
- ENoG for facial nerve integrity (if applicable)

Management
- Establish adequate airway, ensure respiration, and assess circulation.
- Conductive hearing loss may resolve if due to TM trauma or hemotympanum. If persistent at 3 months, consider tympanotomy to assess for sclerosis, ossicular discontinuity, and acquired cholesteatoma.
- Vertigo generally resolves by 6 months, with return of ENG to normal. Acute treatment involves meclizine, promethazine, and diazepam. If it persists, consider a perilymphatic fistula and recommend bed rest, elevation of the head, stool softeners, and antitussives. Surgical repair of the fistula is required if refractory.
- Facial nerve injury should be assessed with ENoG. If there is >90% degeneration within 2 weeks, recommend facial nerve decompression. If delayed-onset or incomplete paralysis occurs, consider observation plus steroids.

- CSF otorrhea may resolve within 2 weeks in most cases with bed rest, head elevation, stool softeners, and lumbar drainage. If it persists, dural repair may be necessary.
- IV antibiotics are indicated if otitis media or meningitis occurs.

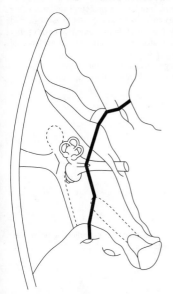

Fig. 15.4 Illustration of transverse temporal bone fracture through the otic capsule.

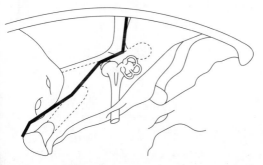

Fig. 15.5 Illustration of longitudinal temporal bone fracture along axis of the petrous ridge.

Complications of surgery

The skull base is an anatomic region of significant complexity through which structures from the brain pass downward to the face and neck and vice versa. The surgeon must have not only a profound understanding of the structural anatomy but also an appreciation for the physiologic and metabolic functions controlled by the region. Improvements in both surgical technique and intraoperative monitoring have reduced the incidence of major surgical morbidity in the region.

Complications of skull base surgery include the following:

- Cranial nerve injury: cranial nerves I–XII are at risk, depending on surgical region
- Vascular complications:
  - Carotid or jugular rupture
  - Vertebral artery rupture
  - Venous thrombosis or thromboembolus
  - Infarction
  - Air embolus
- Cerebral complications
  - Brain edema or herniation
  - Meningitis, intracranial abscess
  - Venous sinus thrombosis
  - Seizures
- CSF leak
- Metabolic alterations: syndrome of inappropriate antidiuretic hormone secretion (SIADH) or diabetes insipidus

Facial plastic surgery and reconstruction

Principles of reconstruction

Head and neck surgery can have devastating functional and cosmetic consequences. Resection of portions of the tongue, palate, pharynx, and larynx can result in severe problems with respiration, deglutition and phonation. Transfacial and transmandibular approaches can result in disfiguring scars as well as impaired function. The basic principles of reconstruction are to restore basic function and physiology, preserve cosmetic subunits, and minimize disfigurement. This can be accomplished in a variety of ways, including the deliberate placement of scars along natural skin creases or along cosmetic subunit boundaries, the restoration of bulk with tissue and filling agents, and sometimes selective facial chemodenervation and reinnervation.

The reconstructive ladder

The reconstructive ladder (Table 16.1) refers to a stepwise approach for the assessment of tissue reconstruction, from the simplest and least invasive to the most invasive and complicated. At the bottom of the ladder is healing by secondary intention, whereas at the top is free flap reconstruction. The approach must be evaluated by considering the functional and cosmetic outcomes of each approach, balanced by the severity of each procedure. Donor site morbidity, patient general medical condition and age, and need for further surgery may all affect the reconstructive algorithm. Reconstruction may also involve the use of obturators and prosthetics. With greater expertise and safety of free flaps, there are many advocates of an escalated reconstruction approach with more aggressive reconstructions for smaller defects.

Table 16.1 Reconstructive ladder

Healing by secondary intention
Primary closure
Skin graft
Local flap based on random blood supply
Local flap based on known local blood supply
Regional flap based on an axial vessel
Free flap reconstruction
Multiple free flap reconstructions

Wound healing

Steps in wound healing

- Step 1: The inflammatory cascade. The break in epithelium and soft tissue damage release inflammatory mediators that activate and recruit fibroblasts. Fibroblasts are activated and begin to migrate into the wound.
- Step 2: The proliferative phase. The fibroblasts produce ground substances (collagen and components of the extracellular matrix) and lay the foundation for epithelial migration and angiogenesis.
- Step 3: The remodeling phase. The collagen and ground substance reorganize to form scar tissue.

Scar revision

Scar revision is based on the excision and redirection of badly healed or badly placed scars into less conspicuous areas. This can be accomplished in several manners; placing scars into natural skin creases, into the margins of cosmetic subunits, and into natural facial shadows. Linear scars tend to be more conspicuous than irregular scars. The most pronounced scars are straight or linear scars that cross multiple subunits, and are perpendicular to natural skin creases. See Figs. 16.1 and 16.2 for common techniques of revising scar.

Relaxed skin tension lines (RSTL)

Skin elasticity is different based on the direction of tension. The RSTLs are the lines of minimal tension of the skin. Incisions should be made parallel to these lines. The lines of maximal extensibility (LME) are perpendicular to the RSTLs. The least skin tension is across the LMEs and will ultimately result in the thinnest scar.

Z-plasty

This is a bilateral transposition and rotational flap that can lengthen, redirect, and reposition scars. Z-plasty is used to reposition scars along RSTLs and to lengthen contracted scars. The angle of the limbs of the Z corresponds to the degree of length added. A 30° angle results in a 25% gain, a 45° angle results in the addition of 50% of length, and 60° angle results in a 75% gain.

M-plasty

The M-plasty is a modification of an elliptical excision with a wedge cut out at each edge. This reduces the length of the scar.

W-plasty and geometric broken line

These techniques are used in an attempt to camouflage linear scars. The original scar is excised and the edges are made into a pattern. A W-shaped pattern is used for W-plasty whereas the geometric broken-line technique uses an irregular pattern.

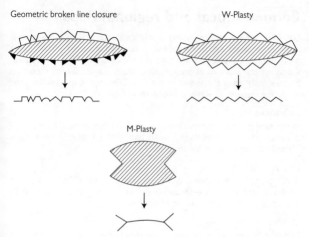

Fig. 16.1 Techniques of scar revision.

Common local and regional flaps

Local flaps have a random blood supply, predominantly from the dermal and subdermal plexus, which are fed by musculocutaneous vessels. In the head and neck, these flaps are quite reliable because of the rich vascular supply of the face. Axial pattern flaps require a consistent superficial blood supply along the length of the flap. These types of flaps are used for reconstruction after skin cancer surgery such as Mohs surgery.

Advancement flaps

In this type of flap linear movement is used to close defects. Examples of advancement type flaps are V-to-Y and bilateral advancement flaps. These are useful around the forehead.

Rotational flaps

This type of flap rotates a flap of tissue into the defect. The incision is a semicircle and requires extensive undermining. The advancement to fill the tissue defect is along the arc of rotation.

Transposition flaps

This type of flap requires tissue elevation and undermining, and the tissue is rotated into the defect, leaving another defect that needs to be closed. Z-plasty, rhomboid flaps, and bilobed flaps are examples of transposition flaps.

Interpolated flaps

These are flaps that use tissue that is elevated with a pedicle and is brought over intact skin bridge. These flaps usually require an axial or named blood supply. An example is the paramedian forehead flap (See Fig. 16.3).

Local flaps

There are many variations of advancement, rotation, and transposition flaps that are used in combinations for reconstruction. There are often multiple types of flaps that can be used for the same defect; the choice is individually tailored for the patient and determined by the surgeon's experience. Table 16.2, and Figs. 16.2 and 16.4 show several examples and illustrations of commonly used superficial skin flaps in the head and neck.

Table 16.2 Superficial skin flaps in the head and neck

Flap	Movement	Common uses
Bilobed flap	R, T, A	Rotates tissue along an axis and directs tension away from the defect. Used commonly around the lateral nose and temple. Main disadvantage is circular scar formation which is difficult to blend and may contract for forming a "pin cushioning" defect.
Rhombic flap	T, R	Highly useful flap. Tension lines and scar direction are highly predictable so that tension can be directed to avoid pulling on adjacent subunits such as eyes and lips. Cheek, lateral nose and temple.
Note flap	T	Lateral nose, small defects

T, transposition; A, advancement; R, rotation.

V to Y advancement flap

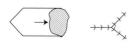

Rotational flap

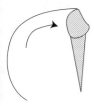

Transpositional flap

Z-Plasty

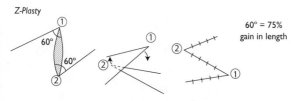

60° = 75% gain in length

Fig. 16.2 Illustration of advancement, rotational, and transposition flaps.

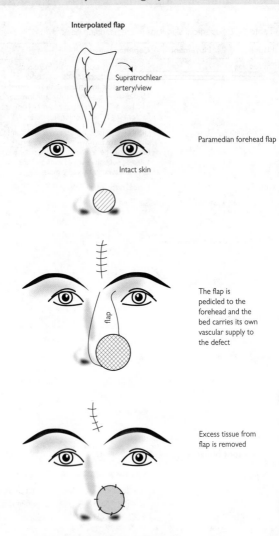

Interpolated flap

Supratrochlear artery/view

Paramedian forehead flap

Intact skin

The flap is pedicled to the forehead and the bed carries its own vascular supply to the defect

flap

Excess tissue from flap is removed

Fig. 16.3 Illustration of an interpolated flap, the paramedian forehead flap.

Pedicled flaps

Pedicled flaps draw nutrition from a large and reliable vascular supply that is usually an axial and named vessel (see Table 16.3). Dissection is performed to carefully preserve this blood supply. The advantage is that the tissue can provide its own vasculature into the tissue defect.

Table 16.3 Pedicled flaps

Flap	Blood supply	Tissue	Common uses
Pectoralis major	Thoracoacromial artery, lateral thoracic artery	M, F, S	Neck and pharynx defects
Sternocleidomastoid	Three arteries: occipital, superior thyroid, thyrocervical trunk	M, F, S	Pharynx and oral cavity
Temporalis	Temporal artery	M	Facial slings and augmentation
Paramedian forehead	Supratrochlear artery	M, S	Nasal reconstruction. See Fig. 16.4

M, muscle; F, fascia; S, skin.

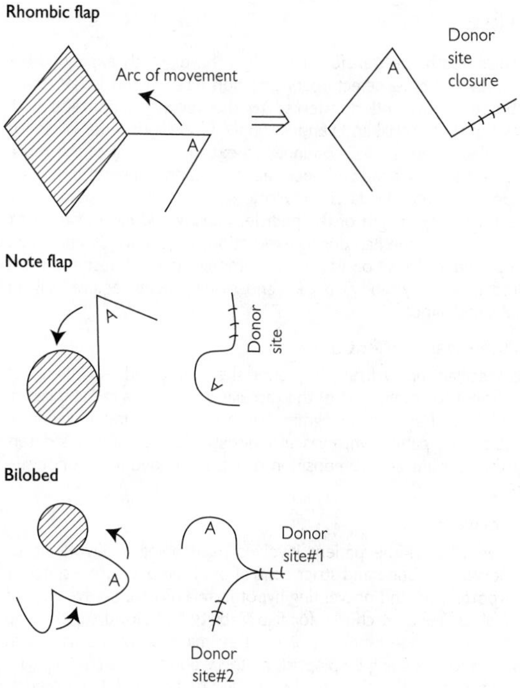

Rhombic flap

Arc of movement

Donor site closure

A

Note flap

Donor site

Bilobed

A

Donor site#1

A

Donor site#2

Fig. 16.4 Illustration of rhombic, note, and bilobed flaps.

Free flaps

Microvascular free tissue transfer or free flaps have greatly expanded the capacity for large tissue defect reconstruction. Free tissue is harvested with its blood supply and transferred to the reconstruction site with anastomosis of the arterial and venous supply. Numerous types of donor flaps are available and the list continues to expand. Several of the more common flaps used for head and neck reconstruction are described here. Flap composition (muscle, fascia, mucosa, skin, nerve, soft tissue, fat), donor site morbidity, length of the pedicle, viability and ease of the flap, and ability to harvest the flap during extirpation surgery are all important factors to consider. These operations are among the lengthiest and most complicated in surgery, and flap care and management require diligent and careful surveillance.

Preoperative assessment

Adequate vascular supply from the donor site is assessed. An Allen test may be sufficient for evaluation of the vascular supply for a radial forearm free flap, while an MRA or angiogram may be necessary for fibular free-flap evaluation in a patient with vascular disease. Choice of flap is determined by the amount and composition of tissue needed and donor site availability.

Postoperative care

Postoperative care of the patient involves maintaining a euvolemic or slightly hypervolemic state and strict control of blood pressure, especially avoiding hypotension, and preventing hypothermia. Postoperative care of the flap involves frequent checks for flap viability and blood supply. Flap monitoring can be done by direct physical examination of the flap, such as observation for bleeding by pinprick and the wound edges and capillary refill. Doppler signals directly over the vascular pedicle and flap temperature are also regularly checked. All of these techniques are used to evaluate flap perfusion. Arterial insufficiency is characterized by a cool, pale appearance and prolonged capillary refill. In vascular insufficiency the flap appears congested and blue, and there is brisk capillary refill along with dark venous blood with pinprick. If there is evidence of anastomotic disruption, surgical exploration should be performed immediately.

The success of free tissue transfer is between 95% and 98%. Problems with the venous system of the flap occur more frequently than those with arterial anastomosis. Most thromboses occur within the first 3 days postoperatively. If there is evidence of flap failure, flap survival depends on the duration of ischemic time before correction. There is a no reflow phenomenon that occurs after a certain ischemic time has elapsed secondary to failure of the microvascular system. Flap salvage rates are between 69% and 100%.

Radial forearm free flap

The radial forearm free flap is one of the most common flaps used in head and neck reconstruction. It is composed primarily of fascia and skin; however, bone and sensory nerve can also be incorporated. The pedicle consists of the radial artery and two venae comitantes. The flap is harvested from the medial surface of the forearm.

The radial forearm free flap has multiple advantages. The vascular pedicle is long, reliable, and readily harvested. It is thin and pliable tissue that can be adapted to a wide variety of different reconstructive needs. The flap can be made sensate by including the medial and lateral antebrachial nerves. The lateral cortex of the distal radius can also be used for bony reconstruction. However, the bone is monocortical and of limited use, as it is quite thin and prone to fracture.

The main drawbacks for the radial forearm free flap involve donor site morbidity. The Allen test is performed preoperatively by checking the perfusion of the hand after digital pressure occlusion of the radial and ulnar arteries. Even with a normal Allen test, however, there is a chance of vascular insufficiency to the hand after removal of the radial artery. In addition, the donor site needs to be covered with a skin graft, which is usually harvested from the thigh.

Fibula free flap

The workhorse for reconstruction of large bony defects is the fibula osteocutaneous free flap. It is excellent for reconstructing mandible and other defects requiring strong, stable bony support. The skin island and accompanying soft tissue are somewhat small and the blood supply to this area is not as robust. The blood supply is based on the peroneal artery, which is a branch of the posterior tibial artery. There is a sensory potential for transfer as well with the lateral sural cutaneous nerve.

A disadvantage of the fibular free flap is variable blood supply and potential donor site morbidity. Patients with peripheral vascular disease are at higher risk for developing ischemic problems with the foot. An intact posterior tibial pulse and dorsal pedalis pulse usually indicate good blood supply. However, vascular studies are commonly performed. An ankle–brachial index of <1 suggests that further study with an arteriogram, duplex, or MRA may be necessary.

Lateral thigh free flap

The lateral thigh free flap is composed of fascia and skin. The blood supply is based on the cutaneous perforators of the deep femoral artery, which originates off the femoral artery. The mass of soft tissue available for harvest can be highly variable depending on body habitus. This soft tissue flap can be used for a wide variety of head and neck reconstructions. In terms of tissue bulk, it is intermediate between the radial forearm and the rectus flaps. Sensory nerve harvest of the lateral femoral cutaneous nerve can also be performed.

Rectus free flap

The rectus myocutaneous free flap is composed of muscle, fascia, fat, and skin. It is substantial flap used to provide bulk for many different types of reconstructions. In the head and neck it can be used for oral cavity, soft tissue, and skull base reconstruction. The blood supply to the pedicle is generally from the deep inferior epigastric vessels, although there is also secondary supply from the deep superior epigastric arteries.

The main advantage of the rectus free flap is its bulk and long vascular pedicle. Because the donor site is away from the head and neck a two-team approach for flap harvest and tumor extirpation can be performed. The most common complications at the donor site include hernias, wound dehiscence, and infection.

Jejunal

The free jejunal flap is composed of a portion of small intestine between the duodenum and the ligament of Treitz. The blood supply is from the jejunal arteries and the associated mesenteric vascular arcades. It is used for reconstruction of mucosal defects within the pharynx or esophagus. Unlike all the other muscular and soft tissue free flaps, the jejunum has peristaltic action. Monitoring of the flap is usually performed by isolating a small segment of the bowel and placing it outside the neck closure.

Principles of aesthetic examination

Principles of aesthetic examination

Beauty is in the eye of the beholder. Because cultural and individual aesthetic sensibility varies, attempts have been made to establish normative values for facial aesthetics, as well as formulas and algorithms to assess and quantify beauty. However, variability is common, and what is a satisfactory outcome for the surgeon may be far from desirable to the patient. Communication and presurgical counseling are paramount prior to any cosmetic undertaking. The use of facial morphing computer programs may help establish realistic goals and expectations. Individual surgeons often have their own sense of aesthetics which are passed on to their treatments.

Generally, an aesthetically pleasing face is smooth, symmetric, proportioned, and balanced. Almost everyone has inherent asymmetries that can be discerned with careful analysis. These asymmetries should be pointed out to patients during preoperative counseling because they may become more obvious after the procedure. Skin texture and facial contour are also important, and initially, less invasive options should be advocated before discussing surgery.

Facial landmarks

The external facial landmarks of the face are illustrated in Fig. 16.5 and listed below (Table 16.4) from superior to inferior. Soft tissue landmarks are determined by facial appearance and can be garnered from facial photographs. Bony landmarks are determined by palpation during the physical examination.

Table 16.4 Facial landmarks

Trichion	Hairline in the mid-sagittal plane
Glabella	On lateral view, most prominent point of the forehead. Usually superior to the root of the nose
Nasion	Deepest point of the nasofrontal angle at the nasofrontal suture line
Radix	Root of the nose
Rhinion	Junction of cartilage and bony nasal dorsum. Bony landmark
Nasal tip	Anterior-most point of the nasal profile
Subnasale	Junction of the columella and philtrum
Stomion	Junction of the upper and lower lips at rest
Pogonion	Anterior border of the chin
Menton	Inferior border of the chin
Cervical point	Junction of the neck and chin

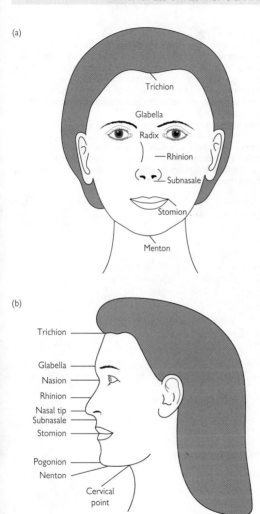

Fig. 16.5(a,b) Facial landmarks.

Facial thirds and fifths

Ideal facial proportions have been the source of debate and scrutiny. Generally, ideal proportions divide the face vertically into thirds and horizontally into fifths. The thirds are from the hairline (trichion) to the glabella, glabella to subnasale, and subnasale to menton. See Figs. 16.6a and b. In the vertical dimension, the width of the eyes, the nose, and distance from the lateral canthus to the lateral projection of the ear are approximately equal.

The *Golden ratio* is a mathematical proportion equal to 1:1.618 (or also 5:8) that is said to have intrinsic harmony. The Golden ratio was celebrated by ancient Greeks and Egyptians and even Leonardo da Vinci as an ideal proportion for beauty. There are several examples of the golden proportion in the face, including the ratio of the length to width of the human head and the ratio of the upper face to mid-face.

(a) Facial thirds

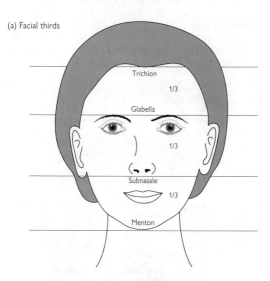

(b) Facial fifths

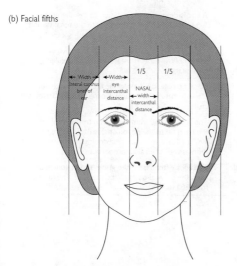

Fig. 16.6(a,b) Facial thirds and facial fifths.

Facial and nasal angles

There have been many methods and algorithms that define the ideal facial angles (see Table 16.5 and Fig. 16.7). The nasafrontal and nasolabial angles are two examples of guidelines that are used frequently during facial analysis.

Table 16.5 Facial and nasal angles

Dorsal line	Line passing through the nasion to the nasal tip
Nasofrontal angle	Angle formed by the line created by the dorsal line of the nose and the line from the nasion to glabella. In men the ideal angle is approximately 115° while in women it is slightly greater, at 120° to 135°.
Nasofacial angle	Incline of the nasal dorsum to the plane of the face; 30° to 40°
Nasolabial	Angles of the lines created by the border of the upper lip and the subnasale and between the subnasale and the columella. The ideal angle in men is approximately 90° and increased in women at 100°–105°. This is reflected by the slightly upturned or rotated appearance in female noses.
Facial plane	The vertical plane passing the through the face at the glabella and pogonion
Goode nasal projection ratio	A line is drawn from the nasion to the alar groove. A perpendicular line is drawn from the nasal tip and the ratio of this line to the nasal length should be 0.55 to 0.60.
Projection	Length of the nose as measured perpendicular to the facial plane
Rotation	Nasal tip rotation is along the arc with the center at the external auditory canal. Corresponds to nasolabial angle
Nasomental	The lines extend from the nasion to the nasal tip, and the nasal tip to the pogonion. Ideal angles are from 120° to 132°. This is used to determine chin-to-nasal tip ratio as well as ideal lip proportions.
Mentocervical	The lines extend from the glabella to pogonion and from the cervical point to the mentum. The ideal is from 80° to 95°.

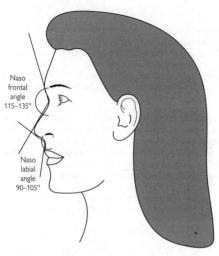

Fig. 16.7 Facial angles.

Photography

Facial photos for aesthetic facial surgery are taken in a standardized and consistent manner. Generally, the facial views are taken with the Frankfort horizontal as the plane of reference. The Frankfort horizontal plane extends from the superior border of the external auditory canal (corresponds to the superior tragus) to the infraorbital rim. Photography for rhinoplasty generally includes frontal, base, lateral, and oblique views.

Rhinoplasty

The nose is at the center of the face and is the focal point. Because it is in the center, the nose sets off many of the other facial features including lips, eyes, cheeks, chin, and forehead. On profile, the nose is the most prominent feature. One of the complexities of rhinoplasty is deciding how an aesthetically harmonious nose can be achieved within the framework of an individual's other features. For instance, increasing nasal projection will soften the features of the chin. A short, rotated nose may look very good in a short individual but inappropriate in someone tall. A cookbook approach to rhinoplasty will ultimately result in unhappy patients.

Nasal anatomy

There are specific terms to describe the different regions of the nose (see Table 16.6). The nose is divided into thirds. The upper third is primarily nasal bone and articulates with the frontal bone. The nasofrontal suture is the groove formed by this articulation and represents the nasion. The region where the upper lateral cartilages overlap with the nasal bones is referred to as the keystone area.

The middle third is composed of the upper lateral cartilages. The upper lateral cartilages are shaped like airplane wings and are attached firmly to the nasal bones. At the caudal edge, they form an interlocking s with the lower lateral cartilages in a region known as the "scroll."

The lower third is composed of the pair of lower lateral cartilages. The lower lateral, or alar, cartilage is shaped like a horseshoe and is divided for reference into three regions: the medial crura, the middle or intermediate crura, and the lateral crura. The structure of the lower lateral cartilages and their attachments to the septum and upper lateral cartilages are the basis for nasal tip support. The internal and external nasal valve areas rely greatly on the cartilaginous support and structure.

Aesthetic assessment

The nose should be approximately one-third the vertical length of the face, beginning at the glabella to subnasale. The width and length should be approximately 0.6 (remember the golden ratio). The width of the nose at the alar base should be approximately the width of the eyes.

Table 16.6 Terminology of nasal landmarks and anatomy

Nasion	Nasofrontal suture line. This usually corresponds to depression at the root of the nose.
Caudal	Towards the tip of the nose
Cephalad	Towards the root of the nose
Scroll area	Refers to the connection of the upper lateral and lower lateral cartilages. The cartilages form an S shape, curling into each other.
Tip	The apex of the lower lateral cartilages at the lateral aspect of the intermediate crus. This is also referred to as the dome.
Supratip break	Region where the tip begins from the dorsum. There is usually a small depression or change in angle.
Keystone area	Area of attachment of the upper lateral cartilages and the nasal bones
Internal nasal valve	Cross-sectional area formed by the caudal edge of the upper lateral cartilages, septum, anterior aspect of the inferior turbinate, and nasal floor. Represents an area of narrowing for nasal airflow. This area is tested by Cottle maneuvers.
External nasal valve	Area formed by the medial and lateral crus of the alar cartilages and nasal floor. Also an area of narrowing. This area is tested by Cottle maneuvers.

Functional assessment

Functional assessment of the nose refers to the ability of the nose to carry and humidify air. Assessment includes the stability of the nasal tip and nasal valves as well as the septum and characteristic of the nasal mucosa. Clinical evaluation for allergies, sinusitis, olfaction, and tear production may be considered. Cottle maneuvers should be performed to assess valve stability and relative contribution to nasal obstruction.

Techniques

There are many different ways to address nasal deformities for aesthetic evaluation, with various techniques available for addressing deformities of the upper, middle, and lower nasal vaults. The tip can be addressed with an *external (open)* approach or an *endonasal (closed)* approach. The open approach allows for direct visualization of the lower lateral cartilages with improved precision and easier assessment for symmetry. An endonasal approach spares the patient an incision across the columella and there is less dissection, resulting in less postoperative swelling. A cartilage delivery method is an endonasal approach that externalizes the lower lateral cartilages. The lower lateral cartilages and nasal tip are altered by shaping and contouring the cartilage and by adding cartilage grafts. Batten grafts are cartilage grafts used to provide additional stability to the intermediate and lateral crura and provide improved stability at the nasal valve. Columellar grafts can be placed to add stability to the nasal tip and alter rotation. Tip grafts can increase nasal projection and alter the appearance of the domes.

The dorsum is composed of both the middle and upper thirds of the nose. There is both cartilage and bone that comprise the dorsum, which need to be addressed separately. Dorsal humps are addressed by resecting cartilage and rasping bone. The middle third can be widened or narrowed by altering the shape of the upper lateral cartilages and by inserting cartilage grafts. Spreader grafts can widen the middle third of the nasal valve. The upper third is generally addressed with osteotomies to correct asymmetries, remove humps, and alter the width.

Complications

Rhinoplasty has several risks. The most common complications are those associated with any surgical procedure, such as bleeding, infection, and unsightly scarring. The unforeseen outcome and/or displeasing aesthetic result is always a possibility and is one reason why patient selection and preoperative counseling are crucial. The surgical approach for rhinoplasty will destabilize the nasal support that needs to be reestablished. There are a variety of named postsurgical deformities, including Polly beak deformity, open roof, pinched nasal appearance, rocker deformity, alar retraction, and columellar show. Valve collapse, vestibular stenosis, and nasal tip instability can result in nasal congestion. Careful preoperative planning and precise surgical technique can minimize these complications.

Rhytidectomy

Treatment of the aging face involves several different approaches. Among the most invasive but most dramatic are operations designed to restore a youthful facial contour and remove excess skin laxity. Rhytidectomy encompasses a group of procedures to reduce facial wrinkles, including neck lift, face lift, and brow lift. Blepharoplasty can also be included and there are numerous modifications in and variations of these procedures.

Anatomy

Fundamental knowledge preceding any discussion of rhytidectomy includes the anatomy and relationships of the skin and fascial tissues within the face and neck. Assessment of the overlying skin for skin damage and photoaging is important. The amount of adipose tissue within the subcutaneous layer will also affect outcome.

The superficial muscular aponeurotic system (SMAS) is a deep fascial layer that envelopes the facial musculature. The SMAS is contiguous with the platysma muscle in the neck and the galea in the forehead. This layer encompasses the superficial temporal fascia as well as the muscles around the mouth and nose and the eyes. Deep to the SMAS lie the parotid fascia, facial nerve, and facial artery. An understanding of this layer is necessary to use deeper planes of dissection for face-lifting, resulting in a more dramatic and longer-lasting operation.

During rhytidectomy, branches of the facial nerve are at risk for damage. Notably, the temporal branch, the zygomatic branch, and the marginal branch may be encountered during dissection along the SMAS.

Assessment

As with any cosmetic procedure, careful patient selection and preoperative assessment are critical. Rhytidectomy is very good at treating the loss of elasticity in the jowls and lower face and excess laxity of the plastysma and fat of the cervical, submental, and submandibular areas. Strong skeletal support and cheek bones tend to favor a good cosmetic outcome. A low-lying hyoid bone will limit the degree of restoration in the neck, as will low-lying submandibular glands.

Types and techniques

Rhytidectomy techniques generally vary depending on the depth of dissection and treatment of the fascial layers. The three general categories of rhytidectomy include the superficial skin lift, the deep plane face-lift, which involves suturing or plication of the SMAS, and even deeper facelifts, which involve multiple fascial approaches and a subperiosteal dissection.

Complications

There are several complications associated with rhytidectomy. The most common are those associated with any surgical procedure—namely, scarring, bleeding, and infection. Other complications include nerve damage. The greater auricular nerve, which provides sensation to the lateral upper neck, lateral face, and ear, is the most commonly injured nerve. There is an approximately 6% rate of injury. The rate of injuries to the motor branches of the facial nerve is approximately 2% to 5%.

Skin resurfacing

There are a variety of effective techniques that can improve skin texture and tone. Mechanical, chemical, and laser- and light-based therapies can eliminate the effects of photodamage and promote neocollagenesis. Skin conditions that can be treated effectively include acne scars, wrinkles, skin discoloration from chronic sun damage, actinic keratoses, scars, and rhinophyma resulting from long-standing rosacea.

Fitzpatrick skin type classification

The Fitzpatrick skin type classification (Table 16.7) is used to grade skin on the basis of response to sun and coloration. The skin type helps predict healing pattern and reactions to inflammation. This is particularly important when determining reaction to dermabrasion, scarring, and laser skin surgery. Darker skin types tend to hyperpigment with inflammation. Laser resurfacing procedures that are safe in pale or white skin may have higher chances of scarring and crusting with darker skin. There are greater risks for hypopigmentation as well with darker skin types.

Table 16.7 Fitzpatrick skin types

Type 1	Pale skin, always burns and never tans
Type 2	White skin, usually burns and tans with difficulty
Type 3	Average tan and sometimes burns
Type 4	Brown or olive skin, tans easily and rarely burns
Type 5	Dark brown skin, always tans, almost never burns
Type 6	Black skin, never burns, always tans

Dermabrasian

Dermabrasion is a mechanical means of removing the epidermis and the papillary dermis. With the use of a rotating wire brush or diamond fraise applied to chilled or tumesced skin, dermabrasion can successfully promote re-epithelialization and reorganize collagen, thereby improving sun-damaged skin. Patients are usually placed on topical tertinoin 0.05% for several weeks prior to treatment. Occlusive dressings may be used after treatment to accelerate wound healing.

Complications of dermabrasion include risk of skin infection, milia, acne flares in people prone to acne, prolonged erythema, and hyper- or hypopigmentation.

Chemical peels

Application of chemical peels is a technique in which a chemical exfoliant is applied to the skin to induce cell turnover and improve skin discoloration and rhytides. Various strengths of acidic and basic chemical agents can produce regenerative changes at superficial to deep levels of the epidermis and dermis. Removal of the stratum corneum (the most superficial layer of the epidermis) is considered a light superficial peel. Destruction of the epidermis is considered a superficial peel and induces epithelial exfoliation and regeneration. Examples of superficial peels include tricholoracetic acid (TCA) 10%–20%, Jessner's solution (a combination of resorcinol, salicylic acid, lactic acid), glycolic acid, salicylic acid (beta-hydroxy), and tretinoin.

Peels that cause additional inflammation within the papillary dermis are considered a medium-depth peel. Examples of medium-depth peels include Jessner's solution, 70% glycolic acid, and solid carbon dioxide with 35% TCA.

Inflammation involving the reticular dermis is considered a deep chemical peel. Examples of deep chemical peels include TCA above 50% or the Gordon-Baker phenol peel. The deeper the peel, the greater the chance for scarring, especially with TCA above 45%. Re-epithelialization typically occurs in 7–10 days in medium and deep peels.

Complications of chemical peels include scarring, prolonged erythema, skin infections, and skin discoloration.

Laser resurfacing

Laser resurfacing involves the use of either a pulsed laser system (usually CO_2 or erbium-YAG (yttrium aluminum garnet) laser for skin ablation. The ultra-pulsed CO_2 laser system (wavelength of 10,600 nm) with a 1000 microsecond pulse duration was one of the first described systems to be used successfully for skin rejuvenation. Multiple CO_2 laser systems are available with a 900–1000 microsecond pulse duration and a computerized scanner to enable systematic treatment of a larger surface area. The erbium-YAG laser (wavelength 2940 nm) produces a more superficial ablation than that of the CO_2 laser system, with less recovery time after treatment.

Another ablative modality that has become available is the use of plasma energy created by highly excited nitrogen gas generated by radiofrequency. Energy levels can vary from less to more ablation depending on the desired result.

Complications from these ablative devices that involve destruction of the superficial skin include skin infection, scarring, prolonged erythema, and hyper- or hypopigmentation.

A recent innovation in the field of laser- and light-based technologies is the concept of fractional resurfacing. Rather than destroying the entire surface of the skin, fractional devices create discrete zones of thermal injury in between intact skin. By leaving islands of normal skin in between wounded skin, rapid re-epithelializatin can occur as early as 24 hours after the procedure. This technique appeals to patients seeking skin rejuvenation who don't want the long recovery period associated with full skin resurfacing. There appear to be fewer side effects associated with this relatively new procedure, as no scarring or long-term hyper- or hypopigmentation has been reported. Erythema typically lasts for 3–4 days after treatment.

Botulinum toxin injections

Botulinum toxin injection for facial rejuvenation is the most common cosmetic procedure performed in the United States. The technique has evolved since its initial applications and is often combined with injectable fillers and laser procedures for optimal facial enhancement. The FDA has approved the cosmetic use of botulinum toxin for the treatment of hyperactive facial lines of the upper face and glabella. Practitioners have used chemical denervation with botulinum toxin for other hyperspastic muscle disorders, autononomic conditions such as hyperhidrosis and drooling, and restoration of facial symmetry for patients with facial synkinesis. There is a growing body of knowledge on the utility of botulinum toxin in the treatment of chronic pain disorders such as headaches and temporomandibular disorders.

Botulinum type A is currently available in the United States as Botox and Reloxin. Botulinum type B is available in the United States as Myobloc. Botox has been FDA approved for the "temporary improvement in the appearance of moderate to severe glabellar lines in adult men and women 65 or younger" since 2002, but its off-label usage is widespread. Reloxin is currently undergoing clinical trials for FDA approval.

The most common cosmetic indications for botulinum toxin include treating the dynamic lines of the upper third of the face such as the glabellar brow furrow, the horizontal frontalis forehead lines, and the periocular crow's feet lines. Other applications of botulinum toxin injections include those to the lower face for perioral rhytides, platysmal banding in the neck, marrionette lines from depressed corners of the mouth, and the "peau d'orange" wrinkling of the chin.

Mechanisms

In 1944, botulinum toxin A was purified in crystalline form, and in the 1950s the mechanism of action was elucidated. By blocking acetylcholine release from motor neurons at the neuromuscular junction, botulinum toxin A enters nerves via protein receptors. The SNARE protein complex is cleaved to inhibit exoctyosis of various neurotransmitters such as acetylcholine. Botulinum toxin A cleaves SNAP-25 whereas type B cleaves vesicle-associated membrane protein (VAMP), also known as synaptobrevin. This process results in an inability to carry out neurotransmitter exocytosis. At the neuromuscular junction, a temporary chemical denervation occurs.

In the early 1970s, botulinum toxin was proposed as a useful agent for treating human strabismus. In 1987, while treating a patient for bepharospasm, a smoothening effect on the glabellar brow furrow was observed. The first description of the cosmetic use of botulinum toxin was published in 1992.

Techniques

The lyophilized powder is usually reconstituted with 1–4.0 ml normal saline, depending on the desired concentration. When 1 ml normal saline is used, the concentration is 100 units/ml. With 2.5 ml normal saline, the final concentration is 40 units/ml. Men usually require more units than women. The common areas of treatment are described in Fig. 16.8.

The glabellar brow furrow can be effectively treated with 20–25 units of Botox, typically placed along five injection points to treat the corrugators and procerus muscle. Four injections are placed on the medial aspect of the brow into the corrugator muscles. Care must be taken to always stay at least 1 cm above the orbital rim along the mid-papillary line to avoid eyelid ptosis. It is helpful to have the patient frown just prior to injection to visualize the corrugators. The fifth injection is placed along the midline of the procerus.

Horizontal forehead lines can be diminished by treating the frontalis. Twelve to 20 units of Botox are usually placed in five to seven divided doses along the forehead. One should try not to inject too inferiorly to avoid causing brow ptosis.

Fine lines in the periorbital region, called "crow's feet," can be diminished with injections of botulinum toxin placed approximately 1 cm lateral to the lateral canthus. A total of 12–15 units on each side is usually injected, divided into three doses. Two to three units may also be injected just below each eye.

For perioral rhytides or smoker's lines, 5–10 units divided into four injections along the orbicularis oris can be administered. Patients should be warned that they may have difficulty with certain actions such as sipping straws or whistling or saying particular sounds.

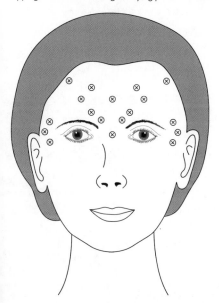

Fig. 16.8 Common areas of botulinum toxin injection.

Common operations

Obtaining informed consent

General principles
The following principles serve as a guideline for the consent process:
- Patients must be given sufficient information—in a way that they can understand—to enable them to exercise their right to make informed decisions about their care.
- Patients' rights are protected by law.
- Effective communication is the key to informed consent.

Consent to investigation and treatment
A doctor who is undertaking a procedure or investigation will need to obtain consent from the patient. When this is not possible, consent can be obtained by a nominated person who is suitably trained and qualified, who understands the risks involved, and who has sufficient knowledge of the proposed investigation or treatment.

It is important that patients make their own decisions about treatment. Ensuring voluntary decision making involves giving the patient a balanced view of the options and explaining the need for informed consent.

Forms of consent
Consent can be either express or implied consent.

Express consent pertains to written or verbally communicated consent in an informed fashion. It must be obtained and documented in the notes when
- the treatment or procedure is complex, or involves significant risks and/or adverse effects;
- there may be significant consequences for the patient's employment or social or personal life;
- the treatment is part of a research program.

Implied consent pertains to consent which is inferred from the patient's actions or other circumstances, even though not expressed in writing. This may include procedures such as an ear examination or in situations where the patient is unconscious, advanced directives or relatives are not found, and life-saving treatment is felt to be in the patient's best interest.

Reviewing consent
Previously obtained consent must be reviewed especially when
- significant time has elapsed between obtaining consent and the start of treatment;
- there have been material changes in the patient's condition, or in any aspects of the proposed treatment plan, which might invalidate the patient's existing consent;
- new, potentially relevant information has become available about the risks of the treatment, for example, or about other treatment options.

Presenting information to patients

Box 17.1 outlines key elements of the informed consent process.

> **Box 17.1 Informed consent process**
>
> - Explain the nature of the decision and procedure.
> - Discuss the risks and benefits and uncertainties of the planned procedure.
> - Provide reasonable alternatives to the procedure, including the option not to treat.
> - Ensure that the patient understands the discussion.
> - Document the acceptance by the patient for the procedure.
> - Give details of the diagnosis and prognosis, including the likely prognosis if the condition is left untreated.

- Answer questions honestly, accurately, and objectively.
- State the purpose of the proposed investigation or treatment, and details of the procedures or therapies involved, including subsidiary treatment such as methods of pain relief.
- Explain the likely benefits and probabilities of success for each option; discuss any serious or frequently occurring risks, including any lifestyle changes that may be necessary as a result of the treatment.
- State how and when the patient's condition and any side effects will be monitored or reassessed.
- Give the name of the doctor who will have overall responsibility for the treatment and, where appropriate, give the names of the senior members of his or her team.
- Remind patients that they can change their mind about a decision at any time and that they have a right to seek a second opinion.
- Where possible, use up-to-date written material and visual and other aids to explain complex aspects of investigation, diagnosis, or treatment.
- Make arrangements to meet particular language and communication needs wherever possible. This could involve translations, independent interpreters, signers, or the patient's representative.
- Be considerate when giving distressing information. Give patients information about counseling services and patient support groups.
- Allow patients sufficient time to reflect on their condition and treatment, before and after making a decision, especially when the information is complex or the risks are serious.

Establishing capacity to make decisions

Fluctuating capacity

Patients who have difficulty retaining information or are only intermittently competent to make a decision should be given assistance to reach an informed decision. Record any decision made while the patient is competent, including the key elements of the consultation. Review these decisions at appropriate intervals before treatment starts, to establish that this decision can be relied on.

Mentally incapacitated patients

If patients lack the capacity to make an informed decision, you may carry out an investigation or treatment that is judged to be in their best interests—including treatment for any mental disorder—provided that they comply with it (see Box 17.2).

Advance statements

Living wills or advance directives must be respected if they are relevant to the current circumstances.

Box 17.2 "Best interests" principle

This involves addressing the following questions:

- Are there any alternative options for treatment or investigation that are clinically indicated?
- Is there any evidence of the patient's previously expressed preferences, including an advance statement?
- What is your own and the health-care team's knowledge of the patient's background, such as cultural, religious, or employment issues?
- What are the views about the patient's preferences given by a third party who may have knowledge of the patient, for example, the patient's partner, family, or caregiver?
- Which option least restricts the patient's future choices, where more than one option (including non-treatment) seems reasonable in the patient's best interest?

Seeking legal counsel

Application to the court may be needed if a patient's capacity to consent is in doubt or if there are differences of opinion over the patient's best interest. This can occur for non-therapeutic or controversial treatments such as organ donation, sterilization or turning off life support.

Tonsillectomy

Indications

- Recurrent acute tonsillitis
- Chronic tonsillitis
- Obstructive sleep apnea (OSA) syndrome
- Oropharyngeal obstruction
- Following one or more peritonsillar abscesses
- Suspected malignancy

Preoperative checks

Examine the pharynx prior to surgery to rule out acute tonsillitis. Discuss the surgery, complications, and the need for time off work or school.

Procedure

Administer endotracheal anesthesia and place patient supine with a bolster under the shoulder and the head supported. This position extends the neck. The nasopharynx is lower than the oropharynx, so blood collects there (Fig. 17.1). Insert and suspend a mouth gag.

The tonsil is grasped with an Allis clamp and retracted medially. Incise the mucosa over the anterior pillar. Dissection is carried to the tonsillar capsule, within a quasi-bloodless plane. The superior pharyngeal constrictor muscle should be kept laterally. The procedure proceeds from superior to inferior where the tonsil approaches the lingual tonsillar tissue. Care must be taken to preserve the posterior tonsillar pillar. Hemostasis of the tonsillar fossa may be achieved using electrocautery or topical hemostatic agents.

Postoperative care

Appropriate pain relief often includes combination acetaminophen and opiate narcotics. One dietary regimen includes clear liquids x 24 hours, then soft foods for 1 week and advance. Monitor the patient for blood loss. Major blood loss is obvious, but minor loss in a young child manifests itself as a rising pulse without increasing pain. Avoid aspirin and NSAIDS.

Complications

- Primary hemorrhage <1%
- Secondary hemorrhage 5%–10%
- Infection
- Dehydration
- Poor pain control

Length of stay

This depends on the unit; the patient may stay in for the day, or overnight.

Discharge advice

Regular analgesia should be taken as the pain often increases around 5 to 7 days after the operation. Give the patient contact details and advice in case of hemorrhage. Patients should stay off work or out of school for 1–2 weeks and avoid strenuous activity for 2 weeks.

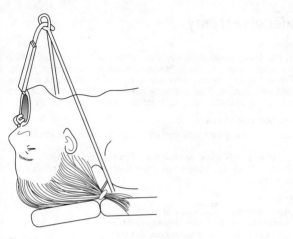

Fig. 17.1 Diagram showing tonsillectomy position.

Adenoidectomy

Indications

Hypertrophic adenoid tissue may obstruct the nasal airway, contributing to snoring, mouth breathing, hyponasal voice, or obstructive apneas. Adenoidal tissue may also contribute to recurrent otitis media or otitis media with effusion. Adenoidectomy may be considered in an adult to obtain biopsy tissue for ruling out infective processes or neoplasms.

Preoperative checks

- Confirm the diagnosis with nasal endoscopy or lateral neck soft tissue X-ray.
- Consider an HIV test in an adult with a hypertrophic adenoid.
- Discuss the surgery, complications, and need for time off work or out of school.

Procedure

- Administer the patient a general anesthetic (GA).
- Position the patient supine with a small shoulder roll.
- Check for bifid uvula or submucous cleft palate.
- Insert and suspend a mouth gag to increase pharyngeal exposure.
- Rubber catheters or a palate elevator can be used as well.
- A nasopharyngeal mirror can be used for direct visualization.
- The adenoid pad may be removed via curette, electrocautery, radiofrequency ablation, or microdebrider.
- Provide hemostasis with cotton gauze pack in the nasopharynx.

Postoperative care

Acetaminophen usually suffices for analgesia. The patient should expect a mildly sore throat. Bleeding is generally minimal.

Complications

Primary hemorrhage is rare, in less than 1% of patients. If it is uncontrolled, examination under anesthesia with cautery may be necessary.

A hypernasal voice (called rhinolalia aperta) may occur if there is velopharyngeal insufficiency (VPI). This complication can severely impact quality of life, especially if nasal regurgitation occurs. Retropharyngeal abscesses may require incision and drainage. Infection should be treated with appropriate antibiotics. Vertebral body subluxation and meningitis are extremely rare yet devastating complications.

Length of stay

An adenoidectomy is generally performed as an outpatient procedure. Patients with OSA who also undergo tonsillectomy should be monitored overnight.

Discharge advice

Most patients will recover rapidly and may require 1 week's rest at home.

Tympanostomy tube insertion

Indications

The patient may present with drum atelectasis, recurrent acute otitis media, and/or persistent middle ear effusion. They may have eustachian tube dysfunction. Rarely, the patient may be undergoing hyperbaric oxygen therapy and cannot equalize pressure.

Preoperative checks

Examine the ear prior to surgery and review the audiogram and tympanometry. Examine the patient's EAC to check access if the operation is being done under local anesthetic.

Procedure

- Use a local or a general anesthetic.
- If a local anesthetic is used, EMLA cream, phenol, or tympanomeatal injection should be instilled under microscope control.
- Using a microscope, insert an ear speculum and identify the antero-inferior segment. Perform a myringotomy using a myringotomy knife. Enough fluid is aspirated to allow the tympanostomy tube to be inserted. The tympanostomy tube is placed through the myringotomy with alligator forceps, and then adjusted with a pick as required.
- If bleeding occurs, use steroid drops to help prevent the tube from occluding.

Postoperative care

Pain is usually minimal and acetaminophen suffices. Topical antibiotic drops may be instilled for a few days postoperatively.

Complications

Occasionally, there may be an infective discharge. Treat this with antibiotic and steroid drops for 1 week. Bleeding from the canal or drum is generally self-limited and topical drops may benefit. The tubes frequently obstruct and may require replacement. Persistent drum perforation is rare, but may necessitate myringoplasty.

Length of stay

This procedure is generally performed in the office (adults) or as ambulatory surgery.

Discharge advice

Many children will swim with tympanostomy tubes in place and have no problem; however, precautions should be taken if discharge follows swimming. Use waterproof earplugs with a swimming cap when bathing. Use similar earplugs for hair washing. Some physicians recommend earplugs anytime the ears may get wet. The initial postoperative visit at 3–4 weeks should be used to document tube patency and obtain an audiogram to determine any change in hearing status.

Tympanoplasty

Indications
- Tympanic membrane perforation
- Severe atelectasis, eustachian tube dysfunction
- Cholesteatoma
- Chronic otitis media

Preoperative care
- Eliminate infection when possible
- Examine patient with the microscope in supine position
- Assess for tympanosclerosis, granulation tissue, cholesteatoma
- Determine status of the scutum and ossicular chain
- Complete audiometric examination
- CT imaging of the temporal bone

Procedure
Anesthetize the patient under GA. Place the head on a ring support with the diseased ear facing upward. The canal is infiltrated with local anesthetic and epinephrine in four quadrants. Clean the ear and prep it with iodine disinfectant. Freshen the perforation edges, then drape the patient.

Either a transcanal or postauricular approach may be employed. Under microscopic guidance, use a canal or round knife to create a flap of canal skin and tympanic membrane. Once elevated, the middle ear can be entered. Cholesteatoma limited to the mesotympanum can be carefully removed. Examine the ossicles for erosion, necrosis, discontinuity, or involvement by cholesteatoma.

Harvest a temporalis fascia graft from the postauricular region, press it and allow it to dry. In the underlay technique, the graft is placed deep to the tympanic membrane. Pack the middle ear with absorbable gelatin foam for the graft to rest upon. Replace the flap along the posterior canal and pack the external ear canal. Close the postauricular incision.

The ossicular chain can be reconstructed with a prosthesis if needed. Tragal cartilage can be used to reconstruct the attic wall.

Postoperative care
The external canal is generally packed with gelatin foam or antibiotic-impregnated gauze. This should be left in place for 6 weeks and removed in the office. An audiogram will be performed at that time. Topical antibiotic drops are unnecessary prior to the 6-week follow-up. The postauricular incision is often closed with subcuticular sutures which does not need to be removed. Steri-strips will fall off in 1–2 weeks.

Complications

- Graft failure with persistent perforation
- Sensorineural or conductive hearing loss
- Postoperative vertigo
- Ear bleeding or infection
- Prosthesis migration or extrusion
- Recurrent cholesteatoma
- Facial nerve injury

Length of stay

This procedure is most often performed on an outpatient basis but patients may be observed overnight, especially if vertigo ensues or if the patient is very young or elderly.

Discharge advice

Patients are instructed not to blow their nose or perform Valsalva maneuvers. The mastoid dressing may be left in place for 48 hours. Hair washing may resume after 72 hours when the postauricular incision is healed, but the ear should be kept dry. The cotton ball at the external meatus should be changed when saturated. The patient should expect a clogged ear until 6 weeks after surgery.

Septoplasty and turbinate reduction

Indications

The patient may present with nasal obstruction or may be having treatment for epistaxis. A bent septum can limit surgical access to the sinuses—a septoplasty may be needed to correct this before sinus surgery. Chronically hypertrophic turbinates may impair nasal airflow. Patients may not respond to appropriate medications (i.e., antihistamines, decongestants, or nasal steroid sprays) or wish to avoid long-term use of these medications.

Preoperative checks

Discuss the surgery, its complications, and the need for time off work with the patient. Examine their ENT system for associated features of rhinitis. Discuss the need for possible continuing treatment for associated rhinitis.

Procedure

Under general anesthesia, place the patient supine on the operating table with the head elevated 30°.

The local anesthetic and epinephrine mixture should be infiltrated into the septum. Approach the septum via a hemitransfixion or Killian incision. Mucoperichondrial flaps should be elevated on both sides of the septum and the cartilage repositioned. Resect gross deviations of cartilage or bone. The 1 cm dorsal and anterior struts should be preserved to keep support. The incision should be sutured. A through-and-through quilting suture may help the flaps adhere.

Infiltrate the turbinates with a local anesthetic. The soft tissue may be reduced using needle point cautery, microdebrider, or radiofrequency energy. Turbinate bone may be resected submucosally if needed. The turbinates may be out fractured to increase cross-sectional area. Alternatively, some surgeons advocate resection of the anterior aspect of the turbinate including soft tissue and bone. Resection of the entire turbinate, although tempting, may result in severe excessive nasal crusting. The nose may be packed if necessary.

Postoperative care

Advise the patient to keep their head up and to avoid blowing their nose for 1 week. The patient may experience nasal crusting and rebound congestion from manipulation. Packs should be removed within 72 hours.

Complications

Epistaxis may occur and might require prolonged packing or cauterization. Septal hematoma will require incision and drainage. Nasal septal perforation may occur from infection, flap trauma, or necrosis.

Length of stay

Most often this procedure is considered ambulatory surgery.

Discharge advice

The patient should avoid strenuous activity for 2 weeks. Nasal toilet with saline sniffs should be performed 4 times a day for 2 weeks.

Direct laryngoscopy

Indications

Direct laryngoscopy involves the use of a rigid laryngoscope, inserted transorally, and advanced to the level of the larynx for viewing laryngeal anatomy. The procedure is indicated for the following:

- Assessing the extent of and performing biopsy of tumors of the laryngopharynx and biopsy
- Evaluating the upper airway following trauma (mechanical or caustic)
- Retrieving foreign bodies
- Excising or ablating benign vocal fold lesions
- Vocal fold augmentation

Preoperative checks

Often the patient will have undergone flexible or indirect laryngoscopy prior to direct laryngoscopy. Educate the patient about local trauma that may follow the insertion of a rigid scope. Dental evaluation with necessary extractions is useful if there are loose teeth. Check for cervical neck range of motion.

Procedure

Place the patient supine in the "sniffing position" with the lower cervical neck slightly flexed and the upper neck extended. The procedure may be performed under general endotracheal, jet ventilation, or spontaneous respiration anesthesia. Once the teeth are protected, advance the laryngoscope through the oral cavity and pharynx posterior to the epiglottis to visualize the larynx. Additional pressure on the anterior neck, at the level of the cricoid cartilage, helps gain additional exposure. The scope may then be suspended on a Mayo stand or suspension apparatus. A microscope may be used for magnification if vocal cord surgery is planned. Biopsies may be obtained using laryngeal biopsy forceps. Once complete, gently remove the scope under direct visualization.

Postoperative care and discharge advice

Patients should be alerted to the possibility of dysphagia and throat pain. If extensive manipulation around the airway was performed, consider IV steroid administration and airway observation in the hospital. Hoarseness may result from local edema, secretions, and vocal fold trauma.

Complications

- Airway obstruction
- Hoarseness (usually transient)
- Hemoptysis
- Aspiration

Length of stay

Depending on the status of the airway, the procedure may be performed on an outpatient basis.

Complications of ear surgery

There are risks with all surgical procedures. The degree of risk is related to both the specific procedure and the underlying pathology. The patient should be given an indication of the likely risk in a sensitive way, so that they are not frightened into abandoning surgery.

A full explanation of the underlying condition will highlight the risks of leaving an ear disease untreated. Risks should be documented in the case notes and on the consent form.

The list of complications for CSOM is similar to that for the operation—the untreated disease carries similar risks to those of the operation. These include the following:

- Hearing loss—temporary and permanent. Always obtain an audiogram at least within 3 months of surgery, but preferably closer to the time of surgery, and perform preoperative tuning fork tests and document your findings.
- Tinnitus—temporary and permanent
- Vertigo or unsteadiness—temporary and permanent
- Facial nerve palsy—temporary and permanent
- Wound infection
- Need for further surgery
- Formation of mastoid cavity with need for ongoing care, e.g., aural toilet

Intraoperative considerations

Many complications can be avoided by taking precautions, e.g., always setting up and checking items such as facial nerve monitors yourself. The precautions taken in the operating room, such as use of a facial nerve monitor, should be recorded on the operation note. Any intraoperative findings or complications should be witnessed and recorded by a senior colleague if available.

Immediate postoperative period

Check for facial nerve palsy in recovery.

Postoperative ward review

Facial nerve function should be checked, along with the eye movements for nystagmus. Weber's tuning fork test should be done. The patient should hear the sound in the operated ear.

Complications of nasal surgery

Nasal surgery includes a large range of procedures on both the external and the internal nose. Procedures on the sinuses are also included.

Complications of external nose surgery

- Imperfect cosmetic result or deformity
- Poor healing of incisions, granuloma, and keloid formation
- Ecchymosis
- Prolonged swelling
- Nasal obstruction
- Dorsal, alar, or tip collapse

Complications of internal nose surgery

- Bleeding and need for packing
- Infection
- Change in nasal shape, e.g., supratip depression with submucous resection (SMR)
- Persistence of nasal blockage for 3 months, or synechia formation
- Need for adjunctive medication.

Complications of sinus surgery

- Bleeding
- Infection
- Orbital damage
- Orbital hematoma
- Optic nerve damage
- CSF leak or intracranial injury

Prevention of complications

Intraoperative considerations

- Good vasoconstriction to maximize vision in operative field and prevent blood loss
- Head-up position to improve venous drainage
- Have preoperative CT scans displayed during surgery to avoid unexpected anatomical variations
- Use of steroids to reduce edema in rhinoplasty
- Swab samples for infected sinus problems

Postoperative problems

- Observation for bleeding—repack if necessary
- Check for orbital hemorrhage
- Check for visual disturbance

Complications of head and neck surgery

These procedures are often prolonged. They can have high morbidity rates and sometimes an associated mortality. The patient group is older and the comorbidities associated with heavy smoking and alcohol abuse make the risks even higher.

Major risks
- Death
- Cardiovascular complications
- Myocardial infarction (MI)
- Deep venous thrombosis (DVT)
- Chest infections
- Pulmonary embolism (PE)
- Flap failure

Preoperative considerations
- Prophylactic antibiotics
- Thromboembolic prophylaxis
- Chest physiotherapy
- Preoperative nutrition—involve dietician
- Smoking cessation
- Admit early for assessment and alcohol detox if necessary

Postoperative considerations
- Continued thromboembolic prophylaxis and early mobilization
- Antibiotics
- Chest physiotherapy
- Balance between analgesia and respiratory depression
- Early removal of central and peripheral lines
- Removal of urinary catheter
- Tracheostomy care
- Pharyngocutaneous fistula care
- Avoidance of pressure sores
- Early action if suspected complication
- Postoperative care on ICU for selected patients
- Nursing protocols and flap observations

Ward care

Preoperative care

Preoperative evaluation

The importance of the preoperative evaluation cannot be understated. Guidelines regarding the extent of preoperative evaluation are institution and physician dependent. Variables taken into consideration include patient age, type and length of surgical procedure planned, anticipated extent of hospitalization, and comorbid medical conditions. In general, patients will undergo preoperative blood testing and clinical examination by a presurgical clinical team or primary care provider. If additional testing is needed, the patient may be sent to a specialist for further medical evaluation.

Institutional directives, aimed at providing cost-effective care, attempt to streamline the preoperative evaluation process. Unnecessary testing raises health-care costs without providing additional medical benefit. However, patient safety is also a primary concern. Surgical morbidity arising from an incomplete preoperative evaluation can be disastrous. The surgeon, anesthesiologist, and preoperative team must work together to promote a safe, cost-effective approach for each patient planned for surgery.

Although no consensus for preoperative screening in routine elective surgery exists, the following list is a proposed guideline for the asymptomatic, healthy patient:

- Hemoglobin level or CBC if excessive blood loss anticipated
- Type and screen/cross-match if excessive blood loss anticipated
- Serum creatinine level for patient age >40
- EKG for patient age >40
- CXR for patient age >60

Additional testing should be ordered on the basis of clinical indicators from the complete history and physical examination. These may include coagulation profile (PT/aPTT), bleeding time, urinalysis, electrolytes, glucose level, liver function tests, echocardiogram, pulmonary function tests, and pregnancy testing in women of child-bearing age.

Special considerations

Deep vein thrombosis (DVT) prophylaxis
The risk of DVT for all surgical patients should be classified as low, medium, or high (see Box 18.1). This is determined by length of surgery, the patient's underlying condition, and past thromboembolic history.

Low	Compression stockings
Medium	Compression stockings + LMW heparin + intraoperative compression boots
High	Stockings + LMW heparin + intraoperative compression boots

---

Box 18.1 Low-molecular-weight (LMW) heparin
(e.g., dalteparin sodium)

Medium risk	2500 U 1–2 hours preoperatively
	2500 U every 24 hours until ambulatory
High risk	2500 U 1–2 hours preoperatively
	5000 U every 24 hours

Antibiotic prophylaxis
Antibiotics may be given to patients with preexisting cardiac problems such as valve insufficiency or for patients who have had major head and neck surgery, to reduce the risk of postoperative infection and fistula formation. Antibiotics should be given within 60 minutes of beginning the procedure. Routine prophylaxis is not required for simple clean wounds, but should be given for clean-contaminated and contaminated wounds.

- Cefazolin 1 g or clindamycin 600–900 mg preoperatively and for 24 hours for skin or oropharyngeal procedures
- Clindamycin 600 mg IV every 8 hours + gentamycin 1.5 mg/kg (check peak and trough serum levels) for broad-spectrum coverage including *Pseudomonas aeruginosa*

Diabetic patients
Diabetic patients should be placed first on the operating list. Non-insulin-dependent patients should avoid oral hypoglycemic agents on the morning of surgery. Insulin-dependent patients may take half the usual morning dose of regular insulin and avoid long-acting formulations on the day of surgery. Take regular finger sticks to monitor sugar level. Use a sliding-scale regular insulin regimen until resuming oral feeds. Table 18.1 gives a common sliding-scale insulin regimen.

Table 18.1 Sliding-scale insulin regimen

For finger stick glucose (g/dL)	Regular insulin dose
0–50	1 amp D50; call MD stat
51–80	Sips of juice
81–200	0 units
201–250	2 units
251–300	4 units
301–350	6 units
351–400	8 units

Postoperative care

Documentation

It is important to document the patient's daily progress and ward round instructions. Any important changes during the day should also be documented. Use a system approach for major head and neck patients, i.e., cardiovascular, pulmonary, renal, nutrition, etc.

Drain care

Monitor suction drainage for each 24-hour period. Remove drains when outputs are less than 30 ml in a 24-hour period, or 10 ml in an 8-hour shift. Strip the drain tubing toward the collection apparatus to remove clots. If the drain loses its vacuum, examine drain position, change the drain bottle for a new one, and consider pressure to the wound or connect the drain to continuous low-pressure wall suction. Prior to removing the drain, take it off suction to avoid injury to underlying structures.

Drains in the neck should be monitored for chyle. This fluid will appear milky and cloud the suction container. Chylous drainage may occur secondary to interruption of the lymphatic vessels or thoracic duct during neck dissection. For leaks <600 ml/day, conservative closed-wound management is initiated. Patients are placed on a medium-chain triglyceride diet if enteral feedings have already begun. Pressure dressings may be applied. If leaks >600 ml/day occur, early wound exploration with hemostatic clip ligation of the leaking vessel is recommended.

Nutrition and fluid balance

Involve a dietician for long-term feeding requirements.

Fluid and electrolytes

Calculate 24-hour maintenance fluid requirements by the patient's weight:
- 0–10 kg   100 ml/kg/24 hours
- 11–20 kg   1000 ml + 50 ml/kg/24 hours
- 20 kg+   1500 ml + 20 ml/kg/24 hours

This volume of fluid requires a composition of 1 mEq of Na^+, 0.5 mEq K^+, and 1.5 mEq Cl^- per kg/24 hours.
- 1 liter normal saline contains 154 mEq of Na^+ and 154 mEq Cl^-.
- 1 liter 1/2 normal saline contains 77 mEq of Na^+ and 77 mEq Cl^-.
- 1 liter lactated ringers contains 130 mEq Na^+, 110 mEq Cl^-, 28 mEq lactate, 4 mEq K^+, and 3 mEq Ca^{2+}.

Maintenance hydration with 5% dextrose in 1/2 normal saline with 20 mEq/L of KCl should avoid sodium overload while replenishing potassium losses. Properly kept fluid balance charts are essential for monitoring the patient's fluid input and output. Record total intake of liquids (enteral and intravenous) and output (urine, drains, oral suction canisters). Pay attention to signs of body fluid excess (edema) and deficit (oliguria, xerostomia).

Nutrition

Postoperative patients require between 40 and 70 kcal/kg/day. Protein requirements range from 1 to 1.5 g/kg/day.

- Fats provide 9 kcal/ gram
- Proteins provide 4 kcal/gram
- Carbohydrates provide 4 kcal/gram

Most ENT patients will be able to be fed via either the mouth or a nasogastric tube (see Boxes 18.2 and 18.3), or by enteral feeding. Patients with severe aspiration or laryngopharyngeal tumors, and patients who have had major head and neck surgery may require gastrostomy tube insertion, especially if a prolonged course is anticipated.

Monitoring intake of calories and other vital substances

- Check weight daily.
- Keep a food record chart.
- Do regular finger stick or urinalysis for glucose.
- Check electrolytes, albumin, and/or prealbumin levels.
- Run vitamins and trace elements screen.

Box 18.2 How to insert a nasogastric tube

- Decongest or anesthetize the nasal cavity.
- Lubricate the tip of the nasogastric tube.
- Have the patient sit upright with the head flexed.
- Advance the tube through the nose parallel to the hard palate.
- Have the patient swallow repeatedly as the tube is advanced down the pharynx.
- Flush port with air and listen for gurgling in stomach; get a low chest X-ray for confirmation if unsure or if tube is to be used for feeding.
- Secure the tube to the nasal ala and dorsum.

Box 18.3 How to unblock a blocked nasogastric tube

- Flush the clear port with water or saline.
- Flush the sump port with air.
- Aspirate tube with an empty syringe.
- Reconnect the tube to low, continuous wall suction.

Postoperative fever

The body's temperature is controlled by the hypothalamus. Fever arises when an alteration in thermoregulatory control causes a temperature set-point elevation. Both infectious and noninfectious causes may alter the temperature set-point.

The febrile patient should undergo a complete history and physical examination. Repeat taking the patient's temperature to confirm fever. Assess all current medications taken, including antibiotics. Examine the surgical wound and surrounding tissues. Listen to the chest, and palpate the abdomen and extremities for tenderness.

On the basis of the examination, obtain cultures from infected sites. Should the cause remain elusive, the following tests should be considered: CBC with differential, urinalysis, chest X-ray, wound, sputum, blood, and catheter tip cultures.

Antipyretics (e.g., acetaminophen) may be useful if the fever is severely elevated, causing patient discomfort. Be aware, however, that antipyretics may mask fever trends. Note that within the first 48–72 hours after surgery, atelectasis ensues, and ambulation or incentive spirometry may resolve the fever. Wound infections generally do not arise until the third or fourth postoperative day. Antibiotic therapy should be tailored according to clinical and microbial assessment. Table 18.2 lists some of the common causes for postoperative fever.

Table 18.2 Causes of postoperative fever

Infectious

- Wound
- Respiratory tract
- Urinary tract
- Meningitis
- Catheter site, phlebitis
- Infected prosthesis

Noninfectious

- Atelectasis
- Malignant hyperthermia
- Venous thrombosis
- Drug or transfusion reaction
- Hyperthyroidism, Addisonian crisis

Care of reconstructive flaps

Reconstructive flaps, either pedicled or transferred as free tissue, are useful to cover large surgical defects in the head and neck. Regional or distant tissues for reconstruction are brought into the defect and vascularized by a pedicle or vessel anastamosis.

It is very important to monitor the viability of these flaps accurately. Often patients are nursed on wards with limited plastic surgery expertise. There is no accepted protocol for postoperative flap care, so discuss specific measures with the surgeon. Immediate intervention may be required if flap failure ensues.

Possible complications

Vascular compromise
- Arterial insufficiency (usually within 24 hours of surgery) manifests as a cool, pale flap that fails to blanch with gentle pressure.
- Venous congestion (develops 48–72 hours postoperatively) presents as a warm, often darker-colored flap that blanches to pressure and bleeds briskly with pinprick.

Hematoma formation necessitates aspiration to prevent necrosis, delayed vascular ingrowth, and infection.

Superficial necrosis/epidermolysis is managed initially by gentle debridement and wet-to-dry dressings.

Infection may require incision and drainage for abscess collection or IV antibiotics for cellulitis.

General principles
- Maintain intravascular volume.
- Maintain adequate hematocrit for oxygen carrying capacity (but not polycythemia).
- Monitor flap appearance by using a flap chart to denote demarcating areas and location of Doppler signal/pedicle.
- Consider antibiotic administration for 24 hours or longer.
- Steroid administration is controversial but may help improve vascular supply by reducing tissue edema.
- Aspirin is usually administered after surgery, once daily.
- Alert reconstructive surgeon immediately if signs of flap failure develop.

Example of hemodynamic goals
- Keep pulse <100
- Maintain systolic BP >100 mmHg
- Keep urine output >35 ml/hr
- Aim for hemoglobin level of 8.5–10.5 g/dl
- If hematocrit <25, give blood

Flap observations
- Direct visualization and assessment of capillary refill with or without needle prick is the most important task.
- A handheld Doppler or Doppler implant may be used to assess blood flow.
- An example of a flap-check schedule may be to assess
  - every 30 min for the first 4 hours, then
  - every hour for the next 48 hours, then
  - every 2 hours for the next 48 hours.

Managing vascular compromise
- Venous congestion
  - Release sutures that may be compromising capillary flow.
  - Serial pinpricks
  - Medicinal leeches
- Arterial insufficiency
  - Mark the flap at the demarcation line.
  - Debride necrotic tissue.
  - Advancement of healthy flap into demarcated areas may help prevent wound contracture.
  - Colloids (i.e., dextran) and anticoagulant benefit unclear
- Hyperbaric oxygen may enhance tissue viability. It may benefit ischemic and congested tissues if available and when instituted early.

Tracheostomy care

The formation of a tracheostomy causes some physiological problems, mainly because it bypasses the nose. The initial requirements of inspired air are humidification, warming, and filtering. After 48 hours the mucous glands in the trachea hypertrophy and help in this process. Tracheostomy care in the early postoperative period centers on avoiding tube obstruction, dislodgement, soft tissue and tracheal infection, and irritation.

Avoiding tracheostomy tube obstruction

- Humidification of inspired air or oxygen
- Soft suction or irrigation of the tracheostomy lumen every 1–2 hours
- Changing the inner cannula each nursing shift

Avoiding tube dislodgment

- Sutures are placed through the flange during surgery, and remain for 1 week. A neck tie or strap provides additional reinforcement.
- Inner cannula changes should be done gently while securing the remainder of the tube in place.
- Agitated patients may need to be restrained or sedated for safety.
- A Bjork flap or stay sutures through tracheal cartilage assist in replacement if accidental dislodgement occurs.
- The tracheostomy site generally "matures" after 1 week.

Avoiding irritation caused by the tube

- The presence of the tube can cause coughing and excess secretion from the bronchopulmonary tree.
- The cuff pressure should be checked routinely to avoid overinflation and tracheal irritation.
- Tracheal irritation can result in a nidus for infection, tracheal erosion, tracheo-innominate fistula, and tracheal stenosis.

Avoiding tracheobronchial infection

- Tracheostomy care should be performed regularly with sterile equipment.
- The tube should be changed first at 1 week postoperatively, and then every 4–6 weeks.
- Purulent material from the wound or tracheal lumen should be sent for culture. Antibiotic therapy may need to be instituted against pathogenic organisms in the sick patient. Note: tubes are often colonized by bacterial flora, which do not necessarily mandate antibiotic administration.

▶ **Important**

Always keep a spare tracheostomy tube, tracheal dilators, inner cannulas, and a suture removal set by the bedside of tracheostomy patients.

Communication with patients and relatives

Patients and relatives may be eager to speak with the surgeon following surgery. Communicating with patients and family causes anxiety in many doctors, as it is not well taught in medical schools and requires the physician to engage in empathetic interpersonal behavior rather than medical or technical prowess.

Basic principles

- Read the patient's notes thoroughly, obtain the facts, and be prepared before any formal talk with a patient or their relatives.
- Anticipate what the involved parties may want to know. Try placing yourself in their position.
- Physically lower yourself to eye level and maintain eye contact throughout the discussion.
- Always speak plainly and honestly.
- Discuss what to expect while in the hospital and thereafter, and provide reassurance that the patient will be well taken care of.

Delivering bad news

Delivering bad news to the patient and family is difficult for most physicians, but having a delineated approach can ease the discomfort for both parties. One such approach is described below.

Establish the setting

- Create an environment conducive to effective communication.
- Ask the patient who they want present, i.e., caregivers.

Determine what the patient knows

- Find out what the patient and family know about the condition.

Determine what the patient wants to know

- Each patient has the right to decline receiving information and designate someone else to act on their behalf.
- Ask whether they want to know the specific details or simply the diagnosis.

Share the news

- Discuss the information in a caring yet straightforward manner.

Respond appropriately to the reaction

- Accept the reaction empathetically and realize that people react to bad news in different ways, i.e. denial, irrational behavior, or silence.

Plan for the next step

- Discuss any additional testing or therapy that will be required.

Discharge planning

Discharging a patient from the hospital following surgery requires thoughtful consideration of many factors. While in the hospital, the patient generally has access to doctors, nursing staff, pain management clinicians, medications, and ancillary supplies to assist with difficulties. Once the patient leaves the hospital, these benefits are discontinued unless specifically ordered and arranged in advance.

Discharge planning should become a coordinated effort between the surgical team, nurses, case manager, and social worker. Planning should begin as soon as the surgery is complete. Despite pressures to discharge patients quickly, the patient must first meet the medical requirements for discharge and all appropriate home care must be arranged.

General points

Consideration of the following questions will help in planning effective discharge.

Meeting discharge criteria
- Are the vital signs and airway stable?
- Is the patient fit to leave—is he or she orientated, mobile, and pain free?
- Is the patient's nutritional support provided for? Have all necessary lines and catheters been removed?
- Is their wound satisfactory?

Medications and supplies
- Does the patient have all necessary medication prescriptions?
- Does the patient require supplemental nutrition?
- If the patient has a tracheostomy, have the necessary suction equipment, tubing, humidification apparatus, care kits, and spare tubes been ordered?
- Does the patient have wound care supplies, e.g., gauze and tape?

Ancillary services
- Does the patient need transport?
- Is a home-care or visiting nurse required?
- Do any medications need monitoring, such as warfarin?
- Does the patient's primary care physician need to know that the patient is leaving the hospital before the discharge letter arrives?

Patient understanding of instructions
- Does the patient understand
  - How to care for the surgical incision?
  - What the limitations are regarding mobility, feeding, and bathing?
  - When he or she may return to school or work?
  - The correct medication regimen to follow?
  - Who to call in case of emergency?
  - When to follow up with the surgeon or other physician?

Practical procedures

How to cauterize the nose

Most nosebleeds originate from the anterior nasal septum at Kiesselbach's plexus. Vessels converge within this site, lying just deep to the nasal mucosa. Exposure to the bleeding site is facilitated with a nasal speculum, headlight, and Fraser suction. Make sure to protect yourself with gloves, a gown, and eye protection. Always ensure that you have performed adequate first-aid steps before attempting to pack or cauterize the nose (see Chapter 20, p. 410). Obtaining a complete blood count and coagulation profile may help identify a platelet or clotting disorder that should be corrected.

Procedure

- Position the patient in the seated upright position.
- Apply one or two cotton buds or a dental roll soaked in 1:10,000 epinephrine and 2% lidocaine, or 4% cocaine solution to the area, and apply pressure for at least 5 minutes.
- Silver nitrate sticks may be applied to the bleeding point for 1 or 2 seconds at a time. Avoid using this form of cautery if the nose is actively bleeding since the blood will simply wash the chemical away. In addition to being ineffective, this will cause unwanted burns to the lip, nose or throat. Instead, wait for the vasoconstrictive effects of the cocaine to work, then apply pressure to the bleeding point. This will nearly always stop the bleeding temporarily before cautery.
- Apply the silver nitrate in a circle starting a few mm from the bleeding point. This will allow any feeding blood vessels to be dealt with prior to cauterizing the main bleeding vessel. A gray eschar should form.
- It may be necessary to reapply the epinephrine or cocaine soaked cotton patty to reduce the bleeding between attempts at cautery. Alternatively, an injection of 1% lidocaine with 1:100,000 epinephrine into the submucoperichondrial plane may decrease bleeding.
- If the nose is still bleeding reapply pressure, and consider packing the nose.
- Electro- or hot wire cautery may be used to good effect in experienced hands.
- If the bleeding site is not immediately obvious, rigid or flexible nasal endoscopy may help.

How to pack the nose

Should cauterization fail to control epistaxis, nasal packing is employed. The goal of nasal packing is to apply pressure to the area of hemorrhage, thereby allowing the body's inherent clotting mechanism to activate. Nasal packs are usually left in place for 24–48 hours. They must be secured anteriorly to prevent them falling back into the airway. Prophylactic antibiotics are often used. Different methods and materials are used to pack the nose.

Always ensure that you have performed adequate first aid steps before attempting to pack or cauterize the nose (see Chapter 20, p. 410).

Anterior nasal packing

Nasal tampons

Nasal tampons are the simplest way to pack the nose (see Fig. 19.1). They consist of a dry sponge, which is placed into the nasal cavity and then hydrated with water or saline. The sponge then dramatically increases in size, compressing the bleeding area. The nasal tampon should be lubricated with an antibiotic ointment prior to insertion. The tip of the nose is lifted and the tampon completely inserted into the nasal cavity, ensuring that it is passed parallel to the floor of the nose. Water or saline is then dripped onto the tampon, which is secured by taping the attached string to the face.

Ribbon gauze packing

Petrolatum-impregnated ribbon gauze may be used to control anterior nosebleeds. Some skill and a good light are needed to place this form of nasal pack effectively. The ribbon is inserted in a layered fashion beginning at the nasal floor and progressing superiorly. The ends of the ribbon should lie externally to prevent ribbon migration posteriorly. Topical analgesia such as lidocaine or cocaine spray is essential prior to packing as this technique may be poorly tolerated by the patient.

Posterior nasal packing

Epistaxis balloon or urinary catheter

A variety of nasal balloons are available (see Fig. 19.2). They are easy to insert and are particularly helpful when the bleeding point is posterior. A Foley urinary catheter is also effective. This is passed into the nasopharynx, inflated, and then pulled anteriorly so that it occludes the posterior choana. It is prevented from slipping back into the nasopharynx or mouth by means of a clamp, which is placed at the nasal vestibule. It is important to put some padding between the skin and a clamp to ensure that no pressure damage is caused. Ribbon gauze may be used to tamponade the anterior nasal cavity and prevent pressure necrosis from the catheter upon the nasal alae.

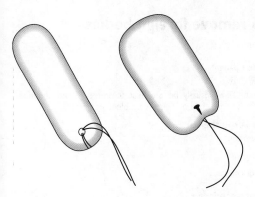

Fig. 19.1 Nasal tampons.

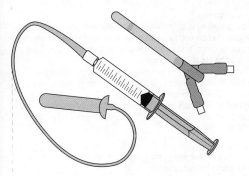

Fig. 19.2 Epistaxis balloons.

How to remove foreign bodies

You will need
- a good light.
- a cooperative patient, and
- good equipment.

The first attempt will usually be the best tolerated. Avoid continued attempts in the anxious child or if significant bleeding occurs.

Foreign bodies in the ear

Signs and symptoms
- Pain
- Hearing loss
- Unilateral discharge
- Bleeding
- May be asymptomatic

Management
- Children will usually require a general anesthetic unless they are remarkably cooperative.
- Insects may be drowned with mineral oil or lidocaine.
- Syringe irrigation may be used if you can be certain there is no trauma to the ear canal or drum. Caution: vegetable material may swell and further obstruct the canal with hydration.
- Use a head lamp or mirror, an operating otoscope or microscope.
- Soft foreign bodies (FB) such as cotton wool may be grasped with a pair of alligator or Tilley's forceps.
- Solid foreign bodies such as a bead are best remove by passing a wax hook or Jobson–Horne probe beyond the foreign body and gently pulling toward you.

Post-procedural care
- Examine the ear canal and assess for a retained FB or trauma to the ear canal or tympanic membrane.
- Apply a single dose of topical antibiotic drops unless a longer course is required for grossly infected ears.
- Perform audiometric examination.
- Instruct the patient to avoid placing foreign bodies, i.e., cotton swabs, in the ear and prevent water from entering the ear if traumatized.

ENT referral
- Refer patient to a specialist if the FB is not easily removed, bleeding ensues, or trauma to the ear canal or tympanic membrane occurs.

Foreign bodies in the nose

Signs and symptoms
- Unilateral foul-smelling discharge
- Unilateral nasal obstruction
- Unilateral vestibulitis
- Epistaxis.

Types of foreign bodies
- Vegetative, i.e., beans, nuts, peas, pits, fruit
- Inanimate, i.e., clay, beads, jewelry, hardware, crayons, erasers
- Alkaline batteries constitute an ENT emergency.
- Rhinoliths are calcified nasal masses resulting from a retained FB for long periods.

Management
- An otoscope can easily be used to examine a child's nose.
- Ask the child to blow their nose if they are able.
- Solid foreign bodies such as beads are best removed by passing a wax hook or Jobson–Horne probe beyond the FB and gently pulling it toward you. Avoid grasping the object with a pair of forceps, since this may simply push it further back into the nose or airway.
- Soft foreign bodies may be grasped and removed with alligator or Tilley's forceps.

ENT referral
- Failed removal
- Excessive bleeding
- Uncooperative child.

Foreign bodies in the throat

See also Esophageal foreign bodies, Chapter 20, p. 422. The cause is often fish or chicken bones.

Signs and symptoms
- Acute onset of symptoms (not days later)
- Constant pricking sensation on every swallow
- Drooling
- Dysphagia
- Localized tenderness in the neck; if above the thyroid cartilage then look carefully in the tongue base and tonsil regions
- Pain on rocking the larynx from side to side
- Soft tissue swelling

Management
- Use a good light to examine the patient.
- Spray the throat with topical anesthetic.
- Try feeling for a FB even if you cannot see one in the tonsil or tongue base.
- Flecks of calcification around the thyroid cartilage are common on X-ray.
- Perform an AP and lateral soft-tissue radiograph of the neck, looking for foreign bodies at the common sites (see Fig. 19.3). Pay particular attention to the following:
  - Tonsil
  - Tongue base/vallecula
  - Posterior pharyngeal wall.
- For foreign bodies not visualized transorally, the patient may be placed supine with a shoulder roll. A Macintosh or Miller laryngoscope can be inserted gently to the vallecula if tolerated. Alternatively, transnasal flexible pharyngoscopy can be used to guide a transoral extraction. These techniques require considerable experience.
- Tilley's forceps are best for removing foreign bodies in the mouth.
- McGill's intubating forceps may be useful for removing foreign bodies in the tongue base or pharynx.

Refer for endoscopy under GA in case of
- Airway compromise—**URGENT**
- Failed removal
- Good history but no FB seen
- X-ray evidence of a FB

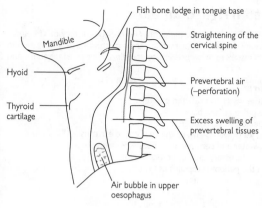

Fig. 19.3 Lateral soft-tissue X-ray of the neck.

How to irrigate an ear

See Fig. 19.4. Check that the patient has no previous history of TM perforation, grommet insertion, or middle ear or mastoid surgery. Irrigation in these circumstances may precipitate middle or inner ear trauma and infection.

Procedure
- Warm the water to body temperature.
- Pull the pinna up and back.
- Use a dedicated ear syringe.
- Aim the jet of water toward the roof of the ear canal.
- Collect water and cerumen into a basin beneath the ear.
- Repeat as necessary until the canal is clear.
- STOP if the patient complains of pain.

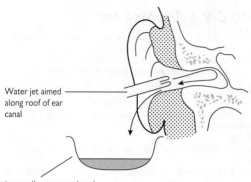

Water jet aimed along roof of ear canal

Basin to collect water, placed under the ear.
Held in position by the patient

Fig. 19.4 How to irrigate an ear.

How to dry a draining ear

Drying an ear with cottonoids should be performed in any ear that is discharging, before topical antibiotics and steroid eardrops are instilled. Since topical antibiotic therapy works by contact, removal of exudate and drainage are necessary to enhance the medication's benefit.

Procedure

- Tease out a clean piece of cotton into a flat sheet
- Twist the cotton onto a suitable carrier such as an orange stick, a Jobson–Horne probe, or even a clean cotton-tipped applicator; see Fig. 19.5.
- Gently rotate the soft end of the cottonoid in the ear canal and remove it.
- Discard the cotton wool and make a new cottonoid—continue until the cotton is returned clean.

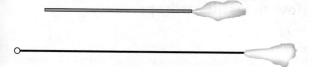

Fig. 19.5 Diagram of a cottonoid for drying a draining ear.

How to instill eardrops

See Fig. 19.6.

Procedure
- Have the patient lie down with the affected ear positioned uppermost.
- Straighten the ear canal by pulling the pinna up and back.
- Squeeze in the appropriate number of drops.
- Use a gentle pumping motion of your finger against the tragus. This will encourage the drops to penetrate into the deep ear canal.
- Have the patient remain with the affected ear upward for at least 10 minutes.
- A cotton ball may be placed at the external meatus.

Consider using an "otowick." This is a preformed sponge and acts as a reservoir, helping to prevent the drops from leaking out of the ear canal. It also serves to reestablish canal patency by expanding against the edematous soft tissue. An otowick is particularly useful in treating otitis externa with severe canal soft-tissue edema with luminal obstruction. It is usually left in place for 48–72 hours prior to removal.

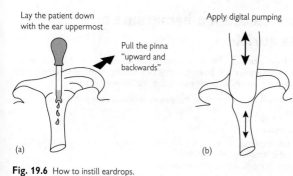

Lay the patient down
with the ear uppermost

Pull the pinna
"upward and
backwards"

Apply digital pumping

(a)

(b)

Fig. 19.6 How to instill eardrops.

How to drain a hematoma of the auricle

This usually occurs after direct trauma to the auricle. It is often caused by a sports injury such as boxing, rugby, or wrestling. If left untreated it may leave a permanent deformity such as a "cauliflower" ear.

Do not neglect the associated head injury that may take priority over the ear injury.

Procedure

- Aspiration may be satisfying, but the collection nearly always reforms, so it is probably best avoided.
- Refer for drainage in sterile conditions.
- Incise the skin of the auricle under local anesthesia in the helical sulcus (see Fig. 19.7).
- Milk out the hematoma.
- The wound may be partially closed and a small rubber band or mini-penrose drain placed.
- Apply pressure to the ear to prevent recollection. Dental rolls or rolled Vaseline gauze may be bolstered to the ear with through-and-through sutures.
- Give antibiotics with appropriate coverage for *S. aureus* and *P. aeruginosa*.
- Reevaluate in 4–5 days.

(a)   (b)

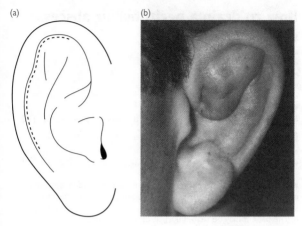

Fig. 19.7 Auricular incision for hematoma evacuation.

How to drain a peritonsillar abscess

Signs and symptoms
- Sore throat—worse on one side
- Pyrexia
- Trismus
- Drooling
- Fetor
- Peritonsillar swelling
- Displacement of the uvula away from the affected side (see Fig. 19.8)

Procedure
- Hydrate patient with IV fluids.
- Administer IV antibiotics with activity against oral gram-positive and anaerobic organisms.
- IV steroid may be administered if trismus prevents adequate exposure.
- Spray the throat with topical anesthetic or inject lidocaine into the mucosa as shown.
- The patient may be seated upright or semi-reclined.
- Have a headlight and suction available.
- Use a 5 ml syringe and a large-bore needle (18 or 20 G) or IV cannula to perform three-point aspiration (see Fig. 19.8).
- Send any pus obtained to microbiology.
- Reserve incision for those cases that recur or fail to resolve within 24 hours.
- Continue antibiotic for 10 days. Have patient gargle with salt water, half-strength peroxide, or oral disinfectant solution.

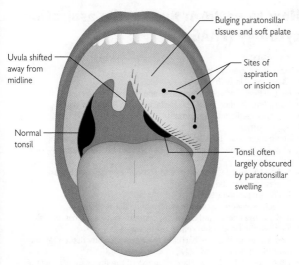

Fig. 19.8 Peristonsillar abscess, incision, and aspiration.

How to perform fine needle aspiration cytology (FNAC)

Procedure

- Have the patient lie down.
- Clean the skin with alcohol.
- Fix the lump between your finger and thumb.
- Use a fine needle (23 or 25G) attached to a 10 ml syringe.
- Pass the needle into the lump.
- Apply suction.
- Move the needle back and forth through the lump using small vibration-type movements—this can prevent contamination by sampling other tissues.
- Make some rotary movements to remove a small core of tissue.
- Release the suction.
- Then remove the needle.
- Detach the needle from the syringe and fill it with air.
- Replace the needle and expel the contents onto a microscope slide.
- Remove the needle and repeat as necessary.
- Check the inside of the barrel of the needle for any tissue that may have become impacted.
- Take a second slide and place it on top of the first, sandwiching the sample between the two.
- Briskly slide the two apart, spreading the sample thinly and evenly.
- Fix and label the slides.
- Apply pressure for 5 minutes and apply a small bandage to the puncture site.

ENT emergencies

Epistaxis

Epistaxis, or a nosebleed, is a common problem that will affect many of us at sometime in our lives. While generally mild and self-limiting, serious sequelae including aspiration, hypotension, and myocardial infarction may occur. To properly care for a nosebleed, the physician should have a solid understanding of the internal nasal anatomy and be familiar with a variety of techniques to control the hemorrhage. The patient is often anxious and frightened and should be properly reassured.

Causes of epistaxis

Local causes
- Nose picking
- Idiopathic
- Trauma (fractures, chemicals, nasogastric tubes)
- Foreign bodies
- Infection
- Tumors

Systemic causes
- Hypertension
- Hepatic and renal failure
- Anticoagulant drugs
- NSAIDs and aspirin
- Coagulopathy (hemophilia, leukemia, DIC, Von Willebrand's disease)
- Hereditary hemorrhagic telangiectasia (an inherited condition with a weakness of the capillary walls leading to vessel fragility)

The anterior aspect of the nasal septum is the most frequent site for bleeding. It has a rich blood supply and a propensity for digital trauma. This part of the nose is known as Little's area (see Fig. 20.1).

First aid for epistaxis
See Fig. 20.2. The patient should be advised to do the following:
- Sit upright with the head extended forward.
- Pinch the fleshy part of the nose (not the bridge) for 10 minutes.
- Avoid swallowing the blood.
- Put an icepack on the nasal bridge.
- Suck an ice cube.

Resuscitation
- Assess blood loss
- Obtain vitals
- Provide oxygen
- Gain intravenous access
- Set up intravenous infusion
- Complete blood count and coagulation profile
- Type and cross-match

See How to cauterize and pack the nose, Chap 19, pp. 390–3.

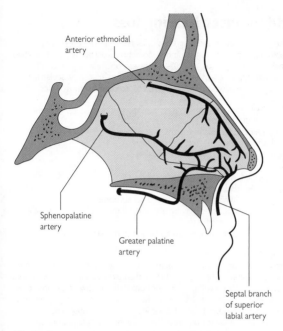

Fig. 20.1 Little's area.

Anterior ethmoidal artery

Sphenopalatine artery

Greater palatine artery

Septal branch of superior labial artery

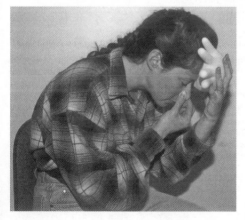

Fig. 20.2 Epistaxis first aid.

Sudden-onset hearing loss

Sudden sensorineural hearing loss (SSNHL) is an ENT emergency. It usually has an acute onset and is sometimes associated with vertigo and balance disturbance. In 90% of cases, one ear alone is affected. The average age of onset is 46–50 years. Viral infections, vascular insults, and autoimmune processes are believed to account for most cases.

Investigations

- Take a full drug history.
- Exclude head or acoustic trauma.
- Check the ear canal to exclude cerumen.
- Check the ear drum to exclude effusion.
- Tuning fork tests:
  - Weber lateralizes to opposite ear
  - Rinne AC>BC in affected ear
- Audiogram confirms hearing loss and no air/bone gap.
- ESR and autoantibodies may be abnormal if there is an autoimmune cause for the hearing loss.
- MRI to exclude acoustic neuroma or other intracranial tumors

Management

The prognosis for recovery depends on many factors. Low- or mid-frequency losses tend to recover better than isolated high-frequency loss. If treatment is initiated within 10 days of onset, the recovery rate improves. If the patient presents within 24–48 hours of onset consider empirical treatment as below, but there is little evidence base to support it:

- Consider admission for bed rest if perilymphatic fistula is suspected.
- Oral steroids (prednisone 1 mg/kg body weight/day)
- Acyclovir or valacyclovir
- Carbogen gas (a mixture of CO_2 and O_2 given for 5 minutes inhalation per waking hour)
- Daily audiograms
- Consider perilymphatic fistula if treatment fails (requires exploration).

If there is any improvement in the hearing at 48 hours, continue with the treatment. If not, discharge patient on a reducing course of prednisone and acyclovir.

- Give a 2-week outpatient assessment and retest the hearing.
- Follow blood and/or MRI results. Consider a hearing aid referral.

Patients presenting to the office with SSNHL are often treated as outpatients. The most common therapeutic trial involves high-dose oral corticosteroids. It is unclear whether antiviral therapy affects outcome. Should the hearing deficit persist following the completion of oral steroids, intratympanic steroid injection should be considered. This procedure may be performed under local anesthesia in the office setting with an operating microscope.

Facial palsy or VII nerve palsy

Paralysis of the facial nerve can be classified by degree (partial or complete), timing of onset (sudden or delayed), and nature (central or peripheral). Causes include traumatic, infectious, neoplastic, congenital, inflammatory, and vascular. The morbidity of facial paralysis can be both cosmetically and functionally disturbing to the patient. A thorough diagnostic workup and management strategy are essential. The House–Brackmann scoring system is frequently used to record the degree of facial weakness (see Box 20.1).

Facial nerve anatomy

The intracranial segment of the facial nerve includes neural pathways from the voluntary motor cortex, internal capsule, extrapyramidal system, midbrain, brainstem, pontine facial nerve nucleus, and cerebellopontine angle (CPA).

The extracranial portion of the nerve is divided into four segments:
- Meatal segment, which travels through the IAC 8 to 10 mm
- Labyrinthine segment, which runs to the geniculate ganglion where the greater superficial petrosal nerve exits
- Tympanic segment, which traverses the middle ear posteriorly to the second genu
- Mastoid segment, which descends inferiorly, gives off the chorda tympani, and exits the stylomastoid foramen

Initial evaluation

- General neurological and cranial nerve exam—to exclude other neurologic deficits
- Exclude serious head injury—fracture of the temporal bone may lead to disruption of the facial nerve in its intratemporal course.
- Examine the ear, looking for cholesteatoma, hemotympanum, middle ear tumor, otomastoiditis, or disruption of the drum or canal.
- Complete audiometric examination
- Check the parotid gland for masses.

Specialized facial nerve testing

Topographic testing

- *Schirmer's test* Evaluates the function of the greater superficial petrosal branch. This test is used to compare tear production of involved and uninvolved eyes.
- *Acoustic reflex test* Evaluates the integrity of the stapedial branch when stimulated by a loud tone. Lesions proximal to this nerve will diminish the stapedial response.

Electrodiagnostic testing

- *Nerve excitability test* Records the minimal amount of current required to produce a noticeable muscular contraction. A difference of 3.5 mAmp between the involved and uninvolved side is significant.

- *Maximal stimulation test* The maximum tolerated current is applied to achieve maximal facial muscle stimulation. The degree of muscle activity is then compared to that of the unaffected side and graded as a percentage, signifying the degree of denervation.
- *Electromyography* Records motor unit potential within facial musculature. Fibrillation potentials may appear within 2–3 weeks after injury and signify denervation. Reinnervation is heralded by the presence of polyphasic potentials that may arise prior to return of facial motion.
- *Electroneurography (ENoG)* Maximal stimulation of facial musculature results in a summation potential whose amplitude is recorded and compared to that of the uninvolved side. The degree of denervation is proportional to the difference in amplitudes between the involved and uninvolved sides.

Causes of lower motor nerve (LMN) facial palsy

- Bell's palsy
- Ramsay Hunt syndrome
- Acute otitis media
- Cholesteatoma
- CPA tumors such as acoustic neuroma
- Trauma
- Parotid gland malignancies
- Sarcoidosis
- Lyme disease, Coxsackie virus, polio, HIV
- Congenital causes (craniofacial anomalies, forceps delivery, infection)

Bell's palsy is probably viral in origin, but the diagnosis is made by excluding the other causes shown above. Starting prednisone (1 mg/kg body weight/day) within 48 hours improves recovery rates. Prognosis is good; 80% of patients fully recover, although return to full function may take months. As with other causes of facial palsy, the failure of complete eye closure can lead to corneal ulceration, so eyedrops or lubricating gel and an eye pad at night may be required. Refer the patient to ophthalmology.

Ramsay Hunt syndrome is due to varicella zoster infection of the facial nerve. The features are similar to those of Bell's palsy with the addition of vesicles on the eardrum, ear canal, pinna, or palate. The affected ear is often extremely painful. Hearing loss and vestibular symptoms may occur. The prognosis is not as good as that for Bell's palsy.

Iatrogenic injury occurs during otologic, parotid, cosmetic, and skull base procedures. During mastoidectomy, the nerve may be injured near the second genu and vertical segment. If transection occurs, a primary neurorrhaphy or interpositional graft should be performed immediately. Postoperatively, if paralysis is immediately noted and nerve integrity unclear, reexploration of the wound is necessary. If onset is delayed, it may be observed and steroid administration considered.

Box 20.1 House–Brackmann grading of facial palsy

I   Normal facial function
II   Slight weakness. Good eye closure, forehead function. Slight oral asymmetry with motion
III Obvious asymmetry and weakness. Complete eye closure with effort. Moderate forehead movement
IV   Obvious asymmetry and weakness. Incomplete eye closure, no forehead motion. Asymmetric mouth with maximum effort
V   Barely perceptible motion. Incomplete eye closure, no forehead motion, slight oral motion
VI   No movement

Periorbital cellulitis

This is a serious and sight-threatening complication of ethmoidal sinusitis. Orbital infections may extend to the orbital apex and cause blindness and intracranial infection. The most common causative organisms include *S. pneumoniae, H. influenza, M. catarrhalis,* and *S. pyogenes* (pediatric). Treatment should be aimed at the underlying sinus infection, although a multidisciplinary team of infectious disease, otolaryngologic, and ophthalmologic specialists is warranted.

Presentation
- Preceding URI with acute sinusitis
- Swelling of the upper lid and periorbital tissues
- Difficulty opening the eye
- Pain around the eye
- Mobility of the globe and visual acuity are unaffected.

Investigations
Look for signs of more severe orbital involvement:
- Proptosis
- Pain on eye movement
- Reduced range of eye movement
- Diplopia
- Change in color vision (red goes first)
- Change in visual acuity.

Management
- Have a high index of suspicion. Obtain a CT scan of the orbits if there is no improvement within 24 hours of starting IV antibiotics.
- Obtain an ophthalmology consultation.
- Take a middle meatal swab for culture.
- Start IV broad-spectrum antibiotics (e.g., ampicillin/sulbactam) with good CSF penetration.
- Any compromise in visual acuity or color vision or suggestion of an intraorbital abscess requires urgent surgical intervention.

If you are treating conservatively, ensure that regular eye observations are performed, as these patients can progress quickly toward blindness.

Orbital complications of sinusitis

The following complications indicate advancing degrees of infection:
Group 1: Preseptal (periorbital) cellulitis
Group 2: Orbital cellulitis
Group 3: Subperiosteal abscess
Group 4: Orbital abscess
Group 5: Cavernous sinus thrombosis

Fractured nose

Any patient with a fractured nose must have sustained a blow or an injury to the head. Direct trauma to the nose or face is usually from a punch, a clash of heads, or a fall. Brisk but short-lived epistaxis is common afterwards.

In patients with a nasal fracture always consider head, cervical spine, and adjacent facial bone injuries.

Investigations

The diagnosis is made on finding a new deformity to the nose, often with associated epistaxis, facial swelling, and periorbital ecchymosis. Ask the patient if their nose has changed shape as a result of their injury. In the first few days after a nasal injury it can be difficult to assess if there is a bony injury because of the degree of associated soft-tissue swelling.

- Try examining the patient from above and behind and looking along the nose from bridge to tip. See Fig. 20.3.
- X-rays are not required to make the diagnosis, but they may be helpful in excluding other bony facial fractures.
- Exclude a septal hematoma by looking for a boggy swelling of the septum, which will cause total or near-total nasal obstruction. This will require urgent treatment by incision and drainage.

Treatment

- Treat any head injury appropriately.
- Administer first aid for epistaxis (see p. 410).
- Consider nasal packing if the bleeding continues (see Chap 19, pp. 392–3).
- Clean and close any overlying skin lacerations.
- Make an ENT outpatient appointment for 5–7 days' time. By then, much of the soft tissue swelling will have resolved, allowing assessment of the bony injury.
- If closed reduction under anesthesia is required, it can be arranged for 7–14 days after the original injury.
- In closed reduction, the nose is packed first with decongestant cottonoids (oxymetazoline, phenylephrine, or cocaine) and the soft tissues around the fracture injected with anesthetic (i.e., 1% lidocaine with epinephrine). The surgeon will elevate the impacted bone and depress the out-fractured bone to reestablish general symmetry. A dorsal nasal splint is then applied.
- Cartilaginous fractures, nasal tip deformities, and septal deviations are generally not addressed during closed reduction. Septorhinoplasty may be considered in some individuals at a later date.

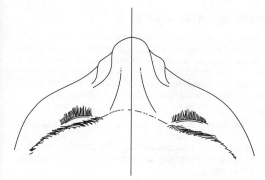

Fig. 20.3 Fractured nose examination (Nasal deformity is best appreciated by examining the patient from above + behind.)

Penetrating neck injury

The otolaryngologist is often called upon to assist in the management of penetrating trauma to the head and neck. Injuries to these areas typically involve either stab wounds, gunshot wounds, or accidental work-related injuries. Depending on the location and mechanism of injury, emergency room personnel, trauma and vascular surgeons, otolaryngologists, anesthesiologists, and interventional radiologists may be summoned.

Anatomy

The neck is often divided into three zones to facilitate risk assessment and decision making (see Fig. 20.4):

- Zone I: Root of the neck to cricoid cartilage. Vital structures include great vessels of the neck and mediastinum, trachea, cervical esophagus, and vertebral artery.
- Zone II: Cricoid cartilage to the angle of the mandible. Risk of injury is to the pharynx, larynx, carotid and vertebral arteries, and jugular vein.
- Zone III: Mandibular angle to skull base. This includes carotid and vertebral arteries, the jugular vein, and cranial nerves.

Presentation

- Injury to vasculature: hematoma, hemorrhage, neurologic deficit, shock
- Injury to the larynx or trachea: airway obstruction, stridor, hoarseness, sucking wound, subcutaneous emphysema
- Injury to the pharyngoesophagus: subcutaneous emphysema, dysphagia, hematemesis

Management

General principles regarding care of the traumatized patient are initiated rapidly.

- **A**irway, **B**reathing, **C**irculation, **D**isability, and **E**xposure represent the order of assessment. (See Chapter 8 for details on the emergency airway.)
- Oxygen and two large-bore IV lines
- Type and cross-match blood
- Cervical neck, lateral, and AP neck soft tissue; chest X-ray films are obtained

Management algorithm by neck zone

Although controversy exists as to the optimal management strategy, the following serves as a useful guide. Any patient with sustained shock or evolving neurologic deficit should undergo immediate neck exploration.

- Zone I injury: Angiography is implemented first. If positive or patient is symptomatic, proceed with neck exploration and laryngoscopy/ esophagoscopy.
- Zone II injury: If patient is symptomatic explore the neck. If asymptomatic, consider angiography, laryngoscopy/ esophagoscopy.
  Explore the neck if guided by findings.
- Zone III injury: Angiography is usually implemented first. If positive or patient is symptomatic, proceed with neck exploration or interventional radiology and laryngoscopy/esophagoscopy (contrast esophagogram).

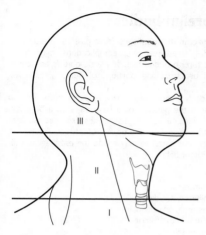

Fig. 20.4 Zones of the neck used for evaluating traumatic injuries.

Esophageal foreign bodies

Foreign bodies often impact in the esophagus. Most pass harmlessly, but hazardous and potentially life-threatening complications may arise. Commonly encountered foreign bodies include plastic objects and coins (pediatric), bones, food products, and portions of dental prostheses (adults).

Sharp foreign bodies carry a much higher risk of perforation. Take a good history to establish if the patient could have ingested a bone or something similar. These include paraesophageal abscess, mediastinitis, airway obstruction, stricture formation, and tracheoesophageal fistula.

Ingested watch or calculator batteries may erode the esophageal wall and must be removed without delay.

Signs and symptoms
- Immediate onset of symptoms
- Early presentation—minutes, not days
- Pain—occasional retrosternal or back pain
- A feeling of an obstruction in the throat
- Drooling or spitting out of saliva
- Point tenderness in the neck
- Pain on rocking the laryngeal skeleton from side to side
- Hemoptysis or hematemesis
- Hoarseness—rare
- Stridor—rare but serious

X-ray findings
See Fig. 19.3.
- Order a plain soft-tissue X-ray of the neck—lateral and AP views.
- Not all bones will show on X-ray, so look for soft tissue swelling in addition to a radio-opaque object.
- Look for an air bubble in the upper esophagus.
- Look for soft tissue swelling of the posterior pharyngeal wall—more than half a vertebral body is abnormal above C4 and more than a whole vertebral body below C4.
- If there is prevertebral air, the esophagus has been perforated.
- Surgical emphysema is a sign of perforation.
- Loss of the normal cervical spine lordosis suggests inflammation of the prevertebral muscles due to an impacted foreign body or an abscess.

Treatment
Endoscopic removal under GA is often required, and is mandatory if there is any suggestion of a sharp foreign body. If the obstruction is a soft bolus, a short period of observation is appropriate with a trial of a carbonated drink (e.g., seltzer) and IV smooth-muscle relaxants.

Following the successful removal of a foreign body, assess for a second foreign body and check for esophageal injury or anatomic obstruction.

Caustic ingestion

The incidence of life-threatening caustic ingestion has decreased over the past century as a result of increased awareness and proper labeling and packaging of household agents. The vast majority of caustic ingestions occur among poorly supervised young children, whereas suicidal attempts and accidental adult ingestions occur less frequently.

The otolaryngologist actively participates in the diagnosis and management of caustic injuries since the upper aerodigestive tract is involved. While most injuries are not immediately life threatening, long-term sequelae, such as esophageal stricture, may seriously impact swallowing function.

Ingested agents fall into two broad categories: caustic agents (alkalis) and corrosive agents (acids). Caustic agents in the form of lye and laundry detergents impart a liquefactive necrosis of tissues with deep penetration. Corrosive materials cause a coagulative necrosis whose depth of penetration is limited by the coagulum. Factors that influence the degree of injury include duration of exposure, concentration, volume consumed, and transit time.

Signs and symptoms
- Oral cavity and pharyngeal burns
- Dysphagia
- Drooling
- Retrosternal or abdominal pain
- Hoarseness or stridor indicate laryngeal involvement with airway obstruction

Management
- Obtain information about agent (name of material, time of ingestion, concentration, immediate first aid).
- Call poison control center hotline.
- Assess ABC's (airway, breathing, circulation).
- Have patient drink water or milk to wash down material.
- Avoid lavage, induced vomiting, or neutralizing agents.
- Consider gastroesophageal endoscopy at 24–48 hours after ingestion.
- Dilute barium swallow may indicate degree of esophageal injury.
- Steroid administration and antibiotics are controversial.
- NPO until esophageal endoscopy confirms degree of injury
- Severe transmural injuries and circumferential involvement may benefit from early esophageal resection with reconstruction.

Complications
- Esophageal perforation with mediastinitis
- Esophageal stricture
- Tracheoesophageal fistula
- Septic shock
- Pneumonia
- Gastric rupture with peritonitis

Secondary tonsillar hemorrhage

Bleeding that occurs 5–10 days after a tonsillectomy operation is known as a secondary tonsillar hemorrhage. (A primary hemorrhage occurs within the first 24 hours after surgery.) A secondary hemorrhage occurs in less than 10% of cases and may result from an infection of the tonsillar fossa, sloughing of the eschar, or trauma. This condition should not be underestimated and patients should be made aware of the possibility of bleeding up to 14 days after surgery.

Common postoperative instructions are aimed at reducing the likelihood of tonsillar bleeding. These typically include the following:
• Clear liquids for 24 hours
• Soft diet for 1–2 weeks
• Avoidance of NSAIDS, aspirin, vitamin E
• Avoidance of exercise or strenuous activity for 2 weeks

Management
• Admit the patient for observation.
• Gain intravenous access.
• Give antibiotics and IV fluids.
• Obtain CBC and coagulation profile.
• Occasionally, cautery may be performed using silver nitrate sticks; however, if significant blood loss occurs, surgical intervention with electrocautery and/or suturing of the tonsillar pillars may be required. Use of GA allows for adequate control of the airway and minimizes aspiration.
• Once controlled, the patient should remain on clear liquids for 24 hours, then advance to soft foods.
• For mild intermittent bleeds, the patient may try gargling with cold water and immediate follow-up in the office for silver nitrate cauterization.

Glossary of ENT terms and eponyms

ABC Airway, breathing, circulation

ABR Auditory brainstem response

ACE Angiotensin converting enzyme

Acoustic neuroma (vestibular schwannoma) A benign tumor of Schwann cell origin arising from the eighth cranial nerve

AE Aryepiglottic

AHI Apnea–Hypopnea Index

Alport syndrome Autosomal dominant disorder consisting of progressive renal failure, sensorineural hearing loss, and maculopathy

ANCA Antinuclear cytoplasmic antibody: positive in Wegener's granulomatosis

Anosmia Loss of the sense of smell

Antrostomy An artificially created opening between the maxillary sinus and nasal cavity

AP Anteroposterior

Arnold's nerve Branch of the vagus to the posterior ear canal and auricle

ASO Antistreptolysin-O

ATLS Advanced trauma life support (protocol)

Avellis syndrome Unilateral paralysis of the soft palate and pharyngolarynx with contralateral loss of pain and temperature sensation to the body

B Bell

BAHA Bone-anchored hearing aid

Barrett's esophagitis Chronic peptic ulceration of the lower esophagus, resulting in columnar metaplasia. Risk of stricture and adenocarcinoma

Basal cell nevus syndrome Autosomal dominant disorder of multiple basal cell epitheliomas with carcinomatous potential, odontogenic keratocyts, palmar pitting, calcification of the falx cerebri, bifid ribs, and frontal bossing

BAWO Bilateral antral washouts

Beckwith-Wiedemann syndrome Macroglossia, gigantism, renal medullary cysts, adrenal cytomegaly, and pancreatic hyperplasia

Behçet syndrome Idiopathic symptom complex of oral and genital ulcers and iritis

Bezold abscess Subperiosteal abscess extending through mastoid cortex along digastric fossa

bid Twice daily

BINA Bilateral intranasal antrostomy

BINP Bilateral intranasal polypectomy

BOR Branchial-oto-renal syndrome. Autosomal disorder of external, middle, or inner ear, plus branchial cleft anomalies and renal dysplasia

Brissaud-Marie syndrome Hysterical unilateral lip and tongue spasm

Broyle's ligament The ligament at the anterior commissure of the larynx

BPPV Benign paroxysmal positional vertigo

BSER Brainstem-evoked response—an objective test of hearing

Cachosmia The sensation of an unpleasant odor

Caloric tests Tests of labyrinthine function in which warm and cool stimuli are imparted to the eardrum

Carhart notch A loss of bone conduction sensitivity at 2–4 kHz in otolsclerosis

CAT Combined approach tympanoplasty

CBC Complete blood count

CEA Carcinoembryonic antigen

Charcot triad Nystagmus, scanning speech, and intention tremor of multiple sclerosis

CHL Conductive hearing loss

Chvostek sign A facial twitch noted upon tapping the skin overlying the intraparotid facial nerve course. May indicate hypocalcemia

CJD Creutzfeldt–Jakob disease

CMV Cytomegalovirus

CN Cranial nerve

Cogan syndrome Autoimmune interstitial keratitis, vertigo, and sensori-neural hearing loss

CPA Cerebellopontine angle

CPAP Continuous positive airway pressure

Crouzon disease (craniofacial dysostosis) Autosomal dominant hyper-telorism, exophthalmos, mandibular hypoplasia and downward-sloping palpebral fissures, parrot-beaked nose, and occasional hearing loss

CSF Cerebrospinal fluid

CSOM Chronic suppurative otitis media

CT Computerized tomography

CVA Cerebrovascular accident

CWD Canal wall down. Tympanomastoid surgery in which the posterior canal wall is removed down to the facial nerve ridge to exteriorize the mastoid. Aka: modified radical mastoidectomy

CWU Canal wall up. A type of tympanomastoid surgery, usually performed for cholesteatoma in which the posterior canal wall is left intact

Dandy syndrome Oscillopsia secondary to bilateral vestibular weakness

dB Decibel

DL Direct laryngoscopy

Dohlman's operation An endoscopic operation on a pharyngeal pouch

DP Direct pharyngoscopy

DVT Deep venous thrombosis

Dysphagia lusoria Compression of the esophagus from an aberrant subclavian artery

EAC External auditory canal

Eagle syndrome Odynophagia secondary to elongation of the styloid process or calcification of the stylohyoid ligament

EAM External auditory meatus

EcoG Echocochleography

EEG Electroencephalography

EKG Electrocardiogram

EMG Electromyography

ENG Electronystagmography

ENoG Electroneurography

ENT Ear, nose, and throat

ESR Erythrocyte sedimentation rate. A nonspecific indicator of an elevated inflammatory response sometimes associated with autoimmune disease

ET Endotrachial

EUA Examination under (general) anesthesia

EUM Examination under the microscope—usually of the ears

FBC Full blood count

FDA U.S. Food and Drug Administration

FDG 18-F-fluorodeoxyglucose

FESS Functional endoscopic sinus surgery

FNAC Fine needle aspiration cytology

Fordyce disease Multiple small, yellowish-white granules along the oral mucosa due to ectopic sebaceous glands

FOSIT Medical shorthand for a feeling of something in the throat

Free flap A surgical reconstructive technique whereby a well-defined flap of tissue (skin ± muscle ± bone) along with its neurovascular pedicle is transferred from donor to recipient site. The blood supply is connected to local blood vessels via microvascular anastomosis. Useful in reconstructing surgical defects following resection of head and neck tumors

Frey syndrome Gustatory sweating, a complication of parotidectomy

FTA-ABS Fluorescent treponemal antibody absorption

GA General anesthesia

GABHS Group A beta-hemolytic streptococcus

Gardner syndrome An autosomal dominant disorder consisting of colonic polyps, epidermal inclusion cysts of the skin, and osteomas of the mandible, maxilla, and long bones

GERD Gastroesophageal reflux disease

GI Gastrointestinal

Globus A sensation of a lump in the throat when on examination no lump can be found (see also FOSIT)

Glottis The region of the larynx at the level of the vocal cords

Glue ear A common cause of conductive hearing loss due to eustachian tube dysfunction. The middle ear fills with thick, sticky fluid, hence its name. Also known as otitis media with effusion (OME) and secretory otitis media (SOM)

Goldenhaar's syndrome A nonhereditary form of hemifacial microsomia with features including underdevelopment of external and middle ear, maxilla, mandible, orbit, facial muscles, and vertebrae

Gradenigo syndrome The onset of retroorbital pain, unilateral otorrhea, and abducens palsy secondary to petrous apicitis

Griesinger sign Mastoid tip edema secondary to septic thrombophlebitis of the sigmoid sinus

Grommet A ventilation tube placed in the eardrum in the treatment of glue ear, also known as tympanostomy tubes or vent tubes

Heerfordt syndrome Uveoparotid fever, a form of sarcoidosis

Hennebert sign Nystagmus produced during pneumatic otoscopy in the absence of a true fistula. Positive in congenital syphilis.

Horner syndrome Ptosis, miosis, and anhidrosis due to cervical sympathetic nerve impairment

HHT Hereditary hemorrhagic telangiectasia, aka Osler-Weber-Rendu syndrome

HIB *Haemophilus influenzae* type B

HME Heat and moisture exchanger

HPV Human papilloma virus, a DNA papovavirus responsible for common warts, laryngeal and sinonasal papillomas, and some squamous cell cancers

HSV Herpes simplex virus

IAC Internal auditory canal

IgE Immunoglobulin E

IJV Internal jugular vein

IM Intramuscular

IV Intravenous

Jacobson's nerve A branch of the glossopharyngeal nerve that traverses the promontory within the middle ear, carrying parasympathetic fibers to the parotid gland

JNA Juvenile nasopharyngeal angiofibroma

Jugular foramen syndrome Paralysis of cranial nerves IX, X, and XI from tumors, adenopathy, or skull base fracture

Kiesselbach plexus The convergence of microvasculature at the anterior nasal septum, aka Little's area

Köerner septum A thin plate of bone separating the mastoid air cells from the antrum

LA Local anesthesia

Large vestibular aqueduct syndrome The enlarged vestibular aqueduct is often an isolated finding in conjunction with ipsilateral sensorineural hearing loss.

LES Lower esophageal sphincter

Lethal midline granuloma A destructive process involving the nasal septum, hard palate, turbinates, and sinuses, now believed to represent a non-Hodgkin's lymphoma

LME Lines of maximal extensibility

LMN Lower motor neuron

LMW Low molecular weight

LTS Laryngotracheal stenosis

Ludwig's angina Infection of the submandibular, sublingual, and submental spaces usually from an odontogenic infection

Marjolin's ulcer An SCC that arises within an old burn scar

MBS Modified barium swallow

Melkersson–Rosenthal syndrome A congenital disease characterized by uni- or bilateral facial paralysis, lip edema, and fissured tongue

Meniere's syndrome Tinnitus, vertigo, aural fullness, and fluctuating hearing loss secondary to endolymphatic hydrops

MI Myocardial infarction

Mikulicz disease Recurrent swelling of the lacrimal and salivary glands

MLB A diagnostic endoscopy. Microlaryngoscopy and bronchoscopy

ML/Microlaryngoscopy Microscopic surgical examination of the larynx using a suspended rigid laryngoscopy and a microscope

MMA Middle meatal antrostomy. A surgical enlargement of the natural maxillary sinus ostium to facilitate ventilation and drainage

Möbius syndrome Congenital paralysis of the facial musculature and abductors of the eye, extremity anomalies, and thoracic muscle aplasia

Mondini malformation Partial aplasia of the membranous and bony inner ear presenting as early-onset hearing loss

MOFIT Multiple out fracture of the inferior turbinate. See also SMD

MRA Magnetic resonance angiogram

MRI Magnetic resonance imaging

MRM Modified radical mastoidectomy. Mastoid surgery performed for cholesteatoma. See CWD.

MRND Modified radical neck dissection. Removal of lymphatic tissue from levels I–V while preserving the spinal accessory nerve, jugular vein, or sternocleidomastoid muscle

MS Multiple sclerosis

MUA Manipulation under anesthesia

NARES Non-allergic rhinitis with eosinophilia

NF2 Neurofibromatosis type 2

NIHL Noise-induced hearing loss

NPC Nasopharyngeal cancer

NSAID Nonsteroidal anti-inflammatory drug

OAE Otoacoustic emissions

OAV Oculoauricular vertebral (syndrome)

Oculopharyngeal syndrome Eyelid ptosis and dysphagia secondary to myopathy. Increased serum creatinine phosphokinase

OE Otitis externa

OME See glue ear

OSA Obstructive sleep apnea

Orbital apex syndrome Compression of neurovascular structures entering the orbit through the superior orbital fissure and optic canal. Paresis of nerves III, IV, V1, and VI is common and vision is impaired by impingement on the optic nerve. May occur from tumors or infection from sinuses

Osteomeatal complex (OMC) The area between the middle turbinate and the lateral nasal wall. The maxillary, frontal, and anterior ethmoid sinuses drain into this area—the final common pathway.

Otorrhea Ear discharge

Panendoscopy (Pan) Laryngoscopy, bronchoscopy, and rigid esophagoscopy are used to evaluate the upper aerodigestive tract. Usually performed to assess malignancy and extent of injury following trauma

PCA Posterior cerebellar artery

PE Pharyngoesophageal; pulmonary embolism

Pec. major Pectoralis major myocutaneous flap. A pedicled flap based on the thoracoacromial artery frequently used to reconstruct surgical defects in the head and neck region

PEG Percutaneous endoscopic gastrostomy

Pendred syndrome An autosomal recessive disorder with bilateral sensorineural hearing loss and thyroid goiter. Positive perchlorate test

PET Positron emission tomography

Pierre Robin syndrome Consists of micrognathia, cleft palate, and glossoptosis. Airway obstruction may warrant tracheostomy.

PND Postnasal drip

PNS Postnasal space

po Per oral (by mouth)

PPI Proton pump inhibitor

Presbycusis The common hearing loss of old age, high frequency, bilateral, and sensorineural in type

PRITs Partial resection of the inferior turbinates. A surgical procedure performed to reduce the nasal obstruction associated with inferior turbinate hypertrophy

prn As needed

Psammoma bodies Calcified concretions seen in papillary thyroid cancer

PSCC Posterior semicircular canal

PTA Pure tone audiogram; pure tone average

PTH Parathyroid hormone

qid Four times daily

Quinsy Peritonsillar abscess

RA Rheumatoid arthritis

Ramsay Hunt syndrome Herpes zoster reactivation of the facial and often vestibulocochlear nerves presenting with facial paralysis, painful vesicles of the ear canal and eardrum, and hearing loss

RAST Radioallergosorbent test

RDI Respiratory Disturbance Index

RERA Respiratory effort-related arousal

Reinke's edema Benign edema of the vocal cords caused by smoking

Rhinorrhea Nasal discharge

RLN Recurrent laryngeal nerve

RPR Rapid plasma reagin

RSTL Relaxed skin tension lines

Samter's triad Allergy sensitivity, nasal polyps, and asthma

SCC Squamous cell carcinoma; semicircular canal

Scheibe aplasia Membranous cochlear and saccular aplasia. The most common form of congenital inner ear malformation. Mondini aplasia is the second most common form.

SDS Speech Discrimination Score

Second look A planned staged operation to ensure that cholesteatoma has not recurred in the mastoid after CWU mastoidectomy

Secretory otitis media (SOM) Glue ear

Serous otitis media (SOM) Glue ear

SGS Subglottic stenosis

SIADH Syndrome of inappropriate antidiuretic hormone secretion

Sjogren syndrome Characterized by dry mouth (xerostomia), dry eyes (keratoconjunctivitis sicca), parotid gland swelling, and arthralgias. Considered an autoimmune disorder. Risk of lymphoma

SLP Speech and language pathologist

SMD Submucus diathermy to the inferior turbinates, performed to reduce the nasal obstruction associated with inferior turbinate hypertrophy

SMR Submucus resection of septum or turbinates

SNHL Sensorineural hearing loss

SOHND Supraomohyoid neck dissection. A type of selective neck dissection to remove nodal tissue in levels I–III of the cervical neck

SRT Speech recognition threshold

T's Tonsils or tonsillectomy

T3 Tri-iodo-thyronine

T4 Thyroxine

TB Tuberculosis

TCA Tricholoacetic acid

TFT Thyroid function test

TGDC Thyroglossal duct cyst

Thornwaldt's cyst A cystic structure protruding into the nasopharyngeal midline believed to result from a remnant of the notochord

TIA Transient ischemic attack

tid Three times daily

TM Tympanic membrane

TMJ Temporomandibular joint

Toxic shock syndrome Multiorgan dysfunction secondary to staphylococcal septicemia. May occur following nasal packing for epistaxis

TSH Thyroid-stimulating hormone

Treacher Collins syndrome (mandibulofacial dysostosis) Characterized by mandibular hypoplasia, downward-slanting palpebral fissure, middle and external ear malformations, and normal IQ

Trousseau sign Carpal spasm induced after tourniquet compression of the arm in hypocalcemic patients

T-tube Long-term grommet

TTS Temporary threshold shift

Tullio phenomenon Vertigo precipitated by loud noise, indicated congenital syphilis, or semicircular canal fistula

Tympanometry The indirect measurement of the middle ear pressure or compliance of the eardrum

Tympanostomy tube A grommet

UARS Upper airway resistance syndrome

U+E Urea + electrolyte

UPP Ulvulopalatoplasty

UPPP Uvulopharyngopalatoplasty

URT Upper respiratory tract

URTI Upper respiratory tract infection

Usher syndrome Autosomal recessive syndrome characterized by visual loss from retinitis pigmentosa, sensorineural hearing loss, and vestibular dysfunction

UV Ultraviolet

VOR Vestibulo-ocular reflux

VPI Velopharyngeal insufficiency

WS Waardenburg syndrome. Autosomal dominant disorder characterized by hypertelorism, flat nasal root, confluent eyebrow, sensorineural hearing loss, white forelock, partial albinism, and multicolored iris

Zellballen Cellular nests surrounded by sustentacular cells found in paraganglioma tumors

Index

Amoxicillin Elixer

Lortab

$\overline{T}_c$ Elixer

$\frac{lbs}{10}$ + 1.2 cc.

po q 4-6 hours (PRN PAIN)

12 oz ∅ Refill

Amoxil

400/5

>10 kg 2.5 ml po bid
>20 kg 5 ml po bid

x's 7 days

Disp # QS
∅ Refills